Topics in Environmental Physiology and Medicine

edited by Karl E. Schaefer

The Influence of Ocular Light Perception on Metabolism in Man and in Animal

F. Hollwich

Translated by Hunter and Hildegarde Hannum

With 59 illustrations

Springer-Verlag   New York   Heidelberg   Berlin

Fritz Hollwich, M.D.
Professor of Ophthalmology
University of Muenster, West Germany
Antonienstrasse 1
8000 München 40
West Germany

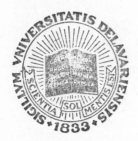

Library of Congress Cataloging in Publication Data

Hollwich, Fritz, 1909–
    The influence of ocular light perception on
metabolism in man and in animal.

    (Topics in environmental physiology and medicine)
    Bibliography: p.
    Includes index.
    1. Light—Physiological effect. 2. Metabolism.
3. Solar radiation—Physiological effect. 4. Eye.
I. Title.
QP82.2.L5H64   591.1'9153   78-17076
ISBN 0-387-90315-1

Printed in the United States of America.

9 8 7 6 5 4 3 2 1

ISBN 0-387-90315-1 Springer-Verlag New York Heidelberg Berlin
ISBN 3-540-90315-1 Springer-Verlag Berlin Heidelberg New York

Preface

This book was written to show that light is a primal element of life. All life originates and develops under the influence of the light of the sun, that "super-terrestrial natural force" (Goethe).

Sunlight influences the vital processes not only of the plant (e.g., heliotropism, photosynthesis) and the animal (e.g., color change, maturation of the gonads) but of man as well. The human organism too reacts "heliotropically," as the 24-hour rhythm of the sleep–waking cycle demonstrates.

Artists have always perceived clearly the intensive stimulatory effect of sunlight on their activity. One is reminded here of Cesare Lombroso, who wrote to his daughter "that thoughts come in the greatest profusion when (my) room is flooded with the sun's rays." Richard Wagner exclaimed: "If only the sun would come out, I would have the score finished in no time." Bernard Shaw had a little cottage where he worked that could be turned according to the position of the sun. The composer Humperdinck wrote: "The sun is indispensable for my work; that is why it is important for me to have my study face east or south."

As these few examples indicate, it is above all those active in the arts who intuitively grasp the positive influence of sunlight on the psycho-physical efficiency of their organism.

In an age, however, when fluorescent lighting turns night into day, we are in danger of forgetting that man is a creature of nature as well as of culture. Artificial light cannot replace natural daylight. As the author was recently able to prove, exposure to bright white artificial illumination of 3,500 lux for a mere 14 days produces a stressful reaction, whereas daylight of the same intensity has a beneficial, vitalizing effect.

In experiments performed over a period of almost three decades (1948–1975), the author and co-workers were the first to demonstrate conclusively that the eye is the channel for light's stimulatory effect. In order to elucidate this effect and separate it clearly from the visual process, in 1948 the author designated the neural pathway conducting the photostimulus to the pituitary gland (hypophysis) as the "energetic portion" of the optic pathway.* Vision itself proceeds independently via the "optic portion" of the optic pathway.

The pages which follow describe a great number of diverse observations and findings concerning the effect of light. In addition, this volume will describe how long it took and what detours had to be made until proof was produced that light's effect on the human organism proceeds, like vision, via the eye.

It is the purpose of this book to demonstrate to architects as well as teachers, physicians, and lighting experts that the source of the light rays entering the eye is of great importance. Artificial light may be an optic substitute but it is by no means equivalent to natural light in physiological terms. Too much artificial fluorescent light interferes with the natural development of the child and subjects the nervous system of the adult to inordinate stress. The health of our organism is dependent to a large degree upon the environmental factor of light, i.e., upon the entry of natural light into the eye.

In retrospect we can say that the introduction of electricity as the energy source for artificial light led to the rise of modern-day civilization: The time had passed when our forebearers went to bed at sunset. Valuable working hours were gained and were utilized to further progress.

When incandescent lamps were still being used, lighting fixtures or lamps were largely an expression of artistic design possessing an atmospheric character, the most impressive example being offered by chandeliers. With the appearance of fluorescent tubes, making inexpensive light available, daylight—which can work like an elixir on bright summer days—was increasingly forced into the background. Light, this "special kind of substance," became a goal in itself.

Classrooms and factories were built with shadowless illumination coming from the ceiling. While it once was a chief task of architecture to introduce daylight into interiors in suitable fashion, this problem no longer exists for the modern architect.

Many of today's large buildings are without windows and are completely air conditioned. Man, who, like all living creatures, evolved under the light of the sun, is thereby cut off not only from visible light but also from the interaction between invisible electromagnetic rays and the earth's electric field.

Previous official specifications for the size and number of windows as entry points for daylight have been altered decisively. Only the so-called "vision windows," i.e., window slits permitting one to look out, are still prescribed in order to counteract the negative psychological effect of the complete exclusion of the outside world. Some buildings have windows which consist of tinted thermopane. During the hot weeks of the year heat is kept out by this means. During the remaining months, however, not only is natural light reduced by 50%, but also—in keeping with the purpose of those windows—daylight's spectrum is considerably reduced, above all in its heat-producing, long-wave red portion. As a result of this decrease in brightness, artificial sources of light with their abbreviated spectrum are turned on much earlier and much more frequently during the day.

In addition, leading lighting engineers have come forward with the assertion that artificial light is equivalent to daylight. To be sure, so-called daylight lamps with their fluorescent tubes emit a bright light which is perfectly adequate for

*See photostimuli to the pineal gland (epiphysis) in Chapter 3.

vision. From morning until evening daylight yields an uneven gradient taking the form of a curve which is relieved by natural shadows, whereas the artificial light of fluorescent tubes emits an even, monotonous, shadowless brightness of linear constancy. The spectrum of artificial light is considerably abbreviated, although there are isolated examples of fluorescent tubes with a spectrum approaching that of daylight. Daylight illuminates places of work from the side; artificial light, on the other hand, illuminates predominantly from the ceiling. The shadowless monotony of artificial light impedes physiologically important adaptive processes of the eye, e.g., pupil response and visual purple regeneration. Bright artificial light entering the eye does intensify the matutinal excretion of cortisol and has an intensely stimulatory effect on the organism. In the course of the day, however, premature fatigue sets in. In addition to this, shadowless brightness impedes the process of accurate spatial vision; metal workers in particular complain about this in their artificially illuminated factories. The more profound effect of protracted intensive artificial light on human metabolism and hormone balance has already been discussed.

In conclusion, to define the crucial issue of today, such an important environmental factor as light must once again be correlated with the needs of man as a creature of nature. Man, in his daily routine, requires the influence of natural environmental factors to a certain degree. Among these are daylight, with its visible and invisible electromagnetic radiation, as well as the unfiltered pure air of the atmosphere and the changing temperature of the external world. Since places of work to a large extent exclude contact with nature, dining and recreation rooms on the premises should be designed to offer a certain compensation. Finally, our homes should also be planned with this purpose in mind. Man, "the Unknown" (Alexis Carrel), has already reached a remarkably high level of civilization in the last decades due to the introduction of many technological options; he should now devote a portion of his energies to the study of those life factors which are indispensable for the maintenance of his health and thus of his existence.

Contents

1
Introduction

Light, like air and water, is a basic element of life. Goethe (1831) called the sun, the dispenser of this light, a "superterrestrial natural force."

In the transition from an aquatic form of life to life on land, our habits and vital functions have adapted themselves to the sun's light in an evolutionary process that has been occurring for millennia. The 24-hour, day–night rhythm regulated the natural course of the day through the changing seasons.

Sunlight has long been recognized as an essential factor along with air and food in the normal development of animals and plants. Mythic depictions by the Egyptians on the stone reliefs of Amarna (14th century B.C.) show the sun's rays as hands enveloping the Pharaoh Ikhnaton and his wife Nefretiti.

Probably the first direct reference in scientific literature to the influence of the sun's light on normal human growth is to be found in Hufeland (1796). In his book *Macrobiotics* he writes:

> Even the human being becomes pale, flabby, and apathetic as a result of being deprived of light, finally losing all his vital energy—as

many a sad example of persons sequestered in a dark dungeon over a long period of time has demonstrated.

In this connection Wimmer (1856), ophthalmologist at the Munich School for the Blind, made a valuable observation:

> The youthful blind person awakens as to new life if we succeed in enabling the eye to perceive light again by removing a cataract or by forming a new pupil.

Investigations into the significance of light for plants go back to the eighteenth century. The fact that they turn toward light (phototropism) was already recognized at that time.

Ott (1964) was the first to show the dependence of leaf movements on light in his skillful time-lapse films. In differentiated experiments, he demonstrated that only the full spectrum of sunlight that has not been reduced by any form of glass induces full growth in plants. Growth and ripening of apples can be retarded, even completely prevented, by filtered light.

Under the influence of the polar winter

(Marx 1946) or after polar expeditions (Gunderson 1969), the participants frequently showed abnormalities in water balance accompanied by edema; general asthenia accompanied by deterioration in behavior; hypotonia; hypoglycemia; sinking of the basal metabolic rate; decrease in potency and libido; loss of hair; insomnia; feelings of oppression, depression, and irritability. These symptoms receded after sufficient exposure to sunlight. Marx designated the light deficiency of the polar winter as the pathogenetic factor in this "hypophysial abnormality."

Jendralski observed a patient in 1951 with cataracts on both lenses and diabetes insipidus with increased excretion of urine due to a pituitary disturbance. When the successful removal of the lenses permitted light to enter both eyes freely, all symptoms disappeared without any further therapeutic measures.

In 1935 the Innsbruck histologist von Schumacher (1939) was struck by the fact that at the Tirolian Hunt Show the number of prizes awarded according to set standards for deer antlers varied from year to year. Schumacher investigated the relevant factors such as snowfall, temperature, and amount of sunshine, coming to the conclusion that the number of hours of sunlight was the most important factor for new growth in the antlers. Thus, the years with the greatest number of hours of sunlight, 1932 and 1933, had the largest number of prize-winning antlers.

According to Schumacher, direct irradiation of the fiber of the newly forming antler is the decisive determinant. We shall return later to this observation, which prompted our own investigations.

Halberg (1953) has the signal honor of having proved experimentally that within the day–night period of 24 hours a so-called circadian rhythm exists in almost all living creatures, with characteristic variations of the vital functions in both phases.

In this connection, observations of people's sensitivity to stimuli or medication at specific times of day are of great empirical significance for medical practice (Sollberger 1965; Halberg 1975). The cardiac patient, for example, responds to diuretics better in the evening than in the morning. The diabetic's morning dose of insulin is more effective the earlier it is administered, the maximum effect occurring around 4 A.M. Some pharmaceutical firms have now begun to produce special medicines taking rhythm into consideration, i.e., for specific times of day. With many diseases there is a tendency for complications to occur at certain times of day. Asthma attacks, acute heart failure, or infarctions most frequently occur around 4 A.M.

The circadian rhythm is likewise of significance in laboratory diagnosis (blood and urinalyses). Thus, almost all serum and urinary metabolites show fluctuations based on the time of day and this must be taken into account in comparative tests.

Daylight per se is consequently a basic element which connects the vital functions occurring in the organism with the natural chronology of the cosmos, as Hufeland expressed it, or with the *Ens astrale,* as Paracelsus put it. With the daily alternation between day and night we participate in the 24-hour circadian (circa diem) rhythmic change from the active diurnal phase to the restorative and regenerative nocturnal one (Halberg 1953).

The question that we will try to answer is how light attains its effect on the human and animal organism. The pages which follow attempt to show that the stimulatory and regulatory effect of light on the human and animal organisms takes place *via the eye.* Independently of the visual process itself ("optic portion" of the visual pathway), light's entry into the eye induces the diencephalic-pituitary system by means of the "energetic portion" (Hollwich 1948) of the visual pathway. In this manner, metabolism and the endocrine system are exposed to the direct influence of light. If these photoimpulses are absent, as is the case with the blind, statistically significant deficiencies occur in both the endocrine and metabolic system.

2

The Energetic Portion of the Optic Nerve

In the popular mind the eye is considered exclusively an organ of vision, and its function consists solely in the perception of visual impressions.

The chamberlike anterior section of the eye (cornea and lens) performs accurate optical transmission; the posterior section (retina) handles the reproduction of objects in the external world. Light, with the visible portion of its spectrum, serves as the medium. In this way a miniature, inverted image of objects in the external world is produced on the retina of both eyes. Conscious perception does not take place, however, until this image is transmitted to the visual center of the brain. For this purpose the sensory cells (cones and rods) of the retina transform the physical stimulus "light" by photochemical means into a neural sensory impulse. The resulting "optic excitations" reach the visual center of the brain via the "optic portion" of the visual pathway, i.e., via the optic nerve, optic chiasm, and optic radiation. Here the visual impressions from both eyes merge: the external object is perceived in the form of a single erect image (Fig. 1).

Along with this optic function the eye performs another intermediary role which has scarcely been recognized up to now but which is no less important for the autonomic (i.e., unconscious) vital functions. Light stimuli entering the eye induce biological functions in the animal and human organism. For this purpose they use separate pathways independent of the visual process. Thus, as a working hypothesis, it seemed practical to distinguish an "energetic" portion of the visual pathway (Hollwich 1948) in contrast to the "optic" portion. This "energetic" portion represents the link between retina and hypothalamus.

Evolutionary History

In terms of evolution there is orginally a close connection between the eye and the hypothalamus. In the area of the diencephalon, the optic vesicle develops on both sides and inverts itself to become a double-walled optic cup (Fig. 2). By means of the optic cup stalk, the retina retains its connection with the diencephalon during the process of further growth as well. Phylogenetically this stalk represents a primitive feature; in the early stages of evolution, it served as an intermediary formation for those fibers which later constituted the optic nerve. This primary connection between the retina and diencephalon is preserved even after formation of the actual "visual pathway." According to Becher (1953), the transmission of photoperception to the vegetative nuclei of the diencephalon is, phylogenetically speaking, the original task of the retina. In contrast to this, "vision" in the strict sense

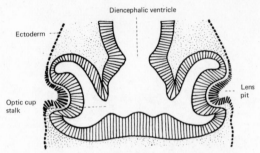

Fig. 2. Origin of the optic cup by inversion of the optic vesicle on the wall of the diencephalon (schematic).

represents a more recent development in terms of evolution. The eye possesses two points of connection: the "optic connection" to the new brain or cerebrum, which does not yet function at birth because the medullary sheath is missing during the first weeks of life; and the connection to the diencephalic-pituitary system, located in the area of the primitive brain, which functions from the very first day of life.

Physiological Findings

The zoologist Mast's experiments in 1916 with the plaice's color adaptations to its environment provided some of the first convincing evidence concerning the effect of light entering the eye: If the plaice's head is put against a dark background, even though the rest of the body is lying against a light background, the fish's body turns dark, and vice versa. The plaice's color adaptation to its background occurs via the eyes (Fig. 3).

The same holds true for color change in the frog (Fig. 4). However, if the animal's eyes are kept shut by suture, as done by Hollwich in 1958, then the color change does not occur; the frog assumes an intermediate shade, neither light nor dark (Fig. 5). Furthermore, the color stimuli of the background have no effect if the optic nerve is severed, the pituitary gland extirpated, or the pituitary stalk cut. This fact led to further experiments to find out whether the color-change stimuli that were perceived by

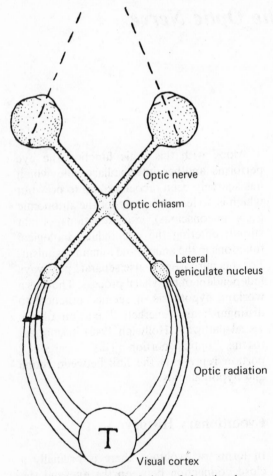

Fig. 1. Schematic depiction of the visual process by a reproduction of a miniature inverted image on the retinas of both eyes. These images merge to form a single erect image, corresponding to the size of the object perceived, on the visual cortex (visual center).

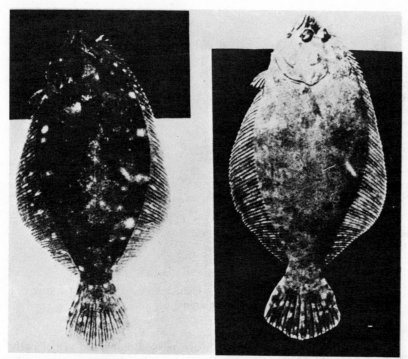

Fig. 3. Color change in the plaice. If the plaice's head is put against a dark background, the fish's body turns dark, even though the rest of the body is lying against a light background; the opposite is also true. The plaice's color adaptation to its background occurs via the eyes.

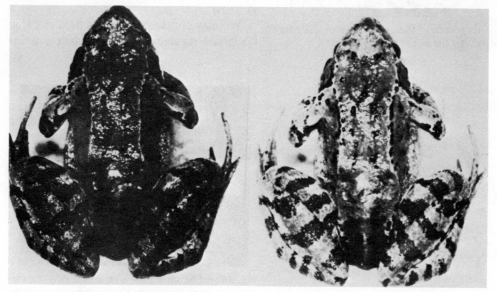

Fig. 4. In a bright environment the frog shows a light skin color (right). In a dark environment the same frog shows a dark skin color (left).

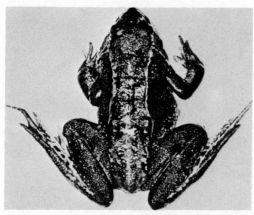

Fig. 5.   The frog assumes an intermediate shade when light's entry into the frog's eye is blocked by suturing its lids.

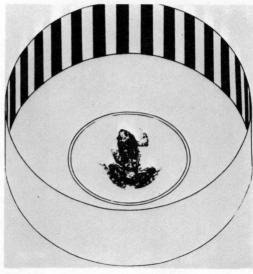

Fig. 8A.   Optokinetic nystagmus of a frog in a revolving drum.

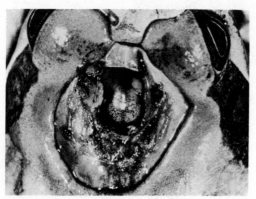

Fig. 6.   Exposure of the optic lobes of the frog by fenestrating the bone of the skull (x6).

the eye were passed along the visual pathway or along special non-optic pathways. To determine this, the frog's visual center was made inoperative by means of electrocoagulation (Figs. 6, 7): vision fails demonstrably in the revolving drum experiment (Figs. 8A, 8B). Nevertheless, the frog's color adaptation to the environment is unimpaired (Figs. 8C, 8D).

We may conclude from this behavior that hormonal regulation of color change is in-

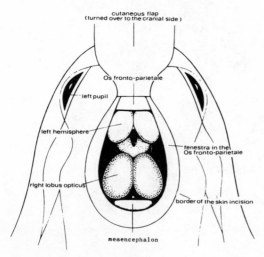

cutaneous flap
(turned over to the cranial side)

Os fronto-parietale

left pupil

left hemisphere

fenestra in the
Os fronto-parietale

right lobus opticus

border of the skin incision

mesencephalon

Fig. 7.   Sketch of Figure 6.

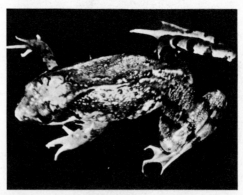

Fig. 8B.   The same frog after destroying the visual center in the brain (lobus opticus on both sides). The frog lost his optokinetic nystagmus by blinding; nevertheless, he is able to change his color.

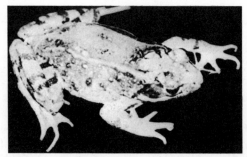

Fig. 8C. This frog's visual centers (lobi optici) have been destroyed by diathermy. In spite of this, the frog exhibits a light skin color on a light background.

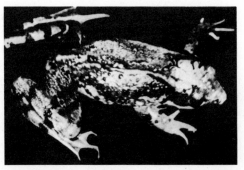

Fig. 8D. The same frog as in Figure 8C takes on a dark skin color when moved from a light to a dark background. Both photographs were taken against the same background. Note the sutures on roof of skull.

duced by photostimuli reaching the pituitary gland via connecting nerves which Hollwich, in a working hypothesis of 1948, described as the "energetic portion" in the visual pathway as opposed to the "optic portion" (Fig. 9).

Clinical and experimental research confirmed this biological effect of ocular light perception on the animal and human organism, i.e., by means of the "energetic portion" of the optic system.

Anatomical Findings

Is there an anatomical substrate for a connection between retina and hypothalamus? Proceeding from Ramón y Cajal's research (1891), Greving was the first (1925) to locate nerve fibers in humans which are not present in the optic tract, but which connect the nervus opticus with the anterior and middle

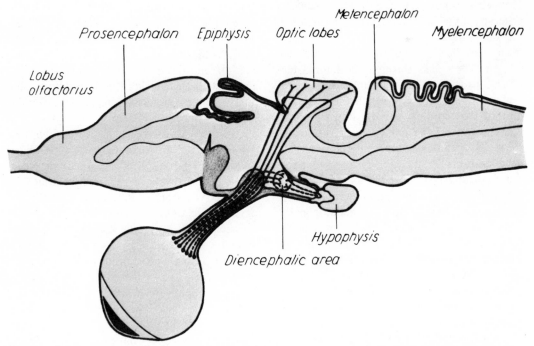

Fig. 9. Schema of the cerebrum of *R. temporaria* (transverse section). Solid line, visual pathway of the optic system; broken line, energetic pathway.

thalamic nuclei. Since these fibers pass through the nucleus supraopticus, Greving suspected the latter's innervation, although he made no further comment about their physiological function. Frey (1935, 1951, 1955) described a "hypothalamic optic root" in the guinea pig: decussate and nondecussate fibers extend from the eye to the central gray matter of the third ventricle. According to Frey, these structures may be identified with the primary optic system. Blind amphibians, for example, demonstrate a connection between retina and optic recess which is still nondecussate. This pathway—the most primitive in phylogenetic terms—can also be found in the dog. Becher (1954, 1955) discovered in the ganglial cellular layer of the third neuron of the retina a smaller variety of cell which is neurosecretory and can be considered a protuberant nucleus of the diencephalon. In his view, these cells are direct receptors for photostimulus and, part of a "heliotropic causal system," they represent the starting point of the vegetative part of the optic system.

Knoche's thorough research (1956, 1957, 1959, 1960) seems to prove the existence of a retino-hypothalamic path. Its fibers utilize the optic nerve as a pathway and depart from the optic chiasm at the ventral superior margin. They pass through the lamina terminalis to the ventral gray matter. A small few of these fibers also reach the posterior lobe of the pituitary via the infundibulum. Knoche proved the existence of this exact route by means of experiments involving degeneration. He used retrograde degeneration to establish the fact that certain cells of the third neuron in the retina were the starting point of the retino-hypothalamic pathway. Likewise, the diencephalon of patients whose eye had had to be removed displayed degenerative atrophy of the retino-hypothalamic pathway.

Carrying forward the word of Becher and Knoche, Blümcke (1958) sought to discover whether a similar fibrous connection of the retina, certain nuclear areas of the hypothalamus, and the pituitary also exists in the guinea pig and the cat. In both animals he too found retino-hypothalamic fibers extending into the autonomic centers of the hypothalamus. By selectively severing the optic nerves, the ciliary vessels, and the ciliary nerves as well as the central artery, Thompson (1951) demonstrated that in the ferret the retina's ganglial cellular layer alone can be responsible for the gonadotropic effect of light. Jefferson (1940) and Hayhow (1959, 1960) doubt the existence of a retino-hypothalamic pathway, since they were not able to locate it in the ferret or in the cat or rat.

In recent years, however, an autoradiographic method has been applied in which radioactively marked amino acids are injected into the posterior chamber of the eye; these are incorporated and metabolized by the retina's ganglial cells and then transported along its axons, especially when neurosecretory ganglial cells are involved. Karlsson and Sjöstrand (1971) investigated this process very carefully, discovering in the rabbit four different and simultaneous rates of transport in the axon and varying rates of assimilation in the lateral geniculate body. The radioactivity can be traced histologically in these anatomical structures. Hendrickson et al (1970, 1972), Moore (1973), Moore and Lenn (1972), Hartwig (1974), and Thorpe and Herbert (1974) all agree with this: Using the autoradiographic method, they report finding a retino-hypothalamic pathway in various mammals and in the house sparrow. The retino-hypothalamic fibers end in the nucleus suprachiasmaticus but in no other hypothalamic structure. There was no indication that the radioactive proteins occurred outside the area of the optic tract or the optic nuclei. Consequently, the radioactivity found in the nucleus suprachiasmaticus can be considered a retinal projection rather than an artifact.

Experiments by Moore and Lenn (1972) support this view. They severed the primary and/or secondary optic pathways without detecting any effect on the adrenal rhythm of the rat; however, when they destroyed the nucleus suprachiasmaticus they discovered that the circadian rhythm was suspended.

Earlier experiments by Moore (1969) indicate that neural connections with the pineal gland also exist. He severed the accessory visual pathways of monkeys, whereupon he observed the effect of added enucleation or prolonged light. In comparison with two groups of monkeys who were not operated on and who showed higher activity of the melatonin (5-methoxy-N-acetyltryptamine)*-synthesizing enzyme *HIOMT* (hydroxy-indole-O-methyltransferase)† in constant brightness than in constant darkness, the animals who were kept in light and who were still able to see although their accessory optic tract had been operated on demonstrated almost half the activity, whereas blind ones showed two-thirds of the

---

*Hormone of the pineal gland that has an effect on the gonads.

†Pacemaking enzyme in the biosynthesis of melatonin; occurs in all body tissue, reaching highest concentration in the pineal organ.

---

enzyme activity of the control group. In the case of both monkey and rat we can assume that the accessory optic system plays a special role in contrast to the other retinal projections; it probably aids in the transmission of neuroendocrine impulses to the pineal gland.

Stephan and Zucker (1972) discovered further indications of a direct role of the nuclei and pathways already described in the regulation of vegetative functions. After the nuclei suprachiasmatici in rats had been made inoperative on both sides by electrolysis, the circadian rhythms regulating their activity and drinking patterns disappeared permanently in spite of their continuing ability to see. We can conclude from this that neurons in these parts of the brain are responsible for eliciting these rhythms and for adapting the organism to changes of light in the environment. The eye fulfills a double function here: owing to the "optic portion" of the visual pathway it receives light for the purpose of visual perception and owing to

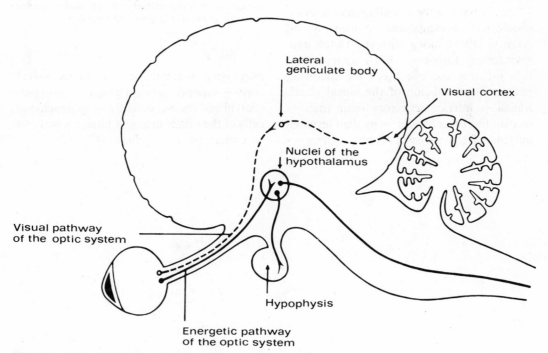

Fig. 10. Schematic graph of the "energetic pathway" (F. Hollwich) of the optic nerve leading from the retina to pituitary gland or hypophysis.

that pathway's "energetic portion" (Hollwich 1948) it transmits light for the purpose
of stimulating the autonomic regulatory centers (Fig. 10).

We know that photostimuli entering the
eye influence the hypothalamus; there is further research which takes into account the
role of the pineal gland (epiphysis cerebri)
here. Browman (1937) demonstrated that
rats exhibit permanent vaginal estrus when
subject to a light of constant intensity. Fiske
et al (1960) observed that the weight of the
pineal gland in rats decreases when they are
exposed to continuous illumination. These
observarions indicate that the pineal gland
contains a substance inhibiting the activity
of the gonads and that the formation or release of this compound decreases when the
animals are kept under conditions of constant light. It was possible to prove, in addition, that the activity of the enzyme
HIOMT, which forms melatonin, depends
significantly upon the intensity of the light to
which the animal is exposed (Wurtman et al
1963, 1964a,b, 1968).

On the basis of these findings and relevant
histological investigations, Wurtmann and
Axelrod (1968), along with the Dutch neu-
roanatomist Kappers (1971), assume that
light entering the eye takes the following
path in its stimulation of the pineal gland:
Retina → inferior accessory optic tract →
median forebrain bundle → median terminal
nucleus of the accessory optic system →

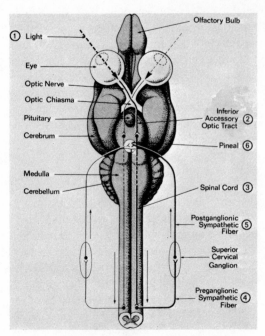

Fig. 11. Schematic diagram of the neural pathway leading from the retina to the pineal gland or
epiphysis (Ep) and possible pathways by which
the pineal gland may act upon the pars distalis of
the hypophysis (Hp) and, via this structure, on
the organs of reproduction. Ht hypothalamus, scg
superior cervical ganglion (Kappers).

preganglial sympathetic tract in the spinal
cord → superior cervical ganglia → postgan-
glial fibers (nerve conarii) → parenchyma
cells of the pineal organ → pituitary body →
secondary hormonal glands (Fig. 11).

3
Light and the Pineal Gland

Almost 300 years ago the French philosopher René Descartes published a drawing showing the optic perception of events, their transference to the brain by means of cords, and the secretion of fluids to the extremities by means of tubes with the aid of the pineal gland (Fig. 12).

The first indication that the pineal organ might play a physiological role was presented by Heubner in 1898. He described the case of a six-year-old boy who demonstrated premature sexual maturity after his pineal gland had been destroyed by a tumor. This led to many experimental attempts to establish the pineal organ's gonadotropic function. Since the classic methods for investigating a secretory gland were applied without taking neural and environmental factors into account, many contradictory results were obtained. Disappointing experiments and the observation that the human pineal gland calcifies in puberty discouraged further study of the organ. Later investigations demonstrated, however, that the calcified pineal gland could nevertheless still be active (Wurtman et al 1964b).

In 1917 zoologists McCord and Allen made a further observation when they found that the skin of frogs and tadpoles rapidly grew paler when they were fed extracts of the pineal glands of cows.

In 1918 the anatomist Holmgren found sensory cells in the pineal region of amphibians and fish that were similar to photo-receptive organelles. As a result of this discovery and of the easily observed, retinalike structure of the pineal organs of lampreys and lizards, the pineal gland was suspected of being a "third eye." Upon removal of the pineal eye of lampreys it turned out that these animals no longer grew pale when placed in the dark (Young 1935). Later, Kelly's investigations with an electron microscope (1962) showed a surprising similarity between the photoreceptive cells of the pineal organ of the frog and those of the frog's retina. At approximately the same time, the neurophysiologists Dodt and Heerd (1962) demonstrated that the pineal organ of the frog can convert light of various wavelengths into neural impulses.

But it was not until 1958 that the biochemist and dermatologist A.B. Lerner was able to isolate the active element in the pi-

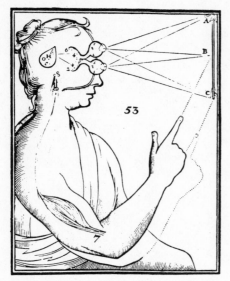

Fig. 12. Reproduction of Descartes' drawing showing the optic perception of events, their transference to the brain by means of cords, and the secretion of fluids to the extremities by means of tubes with the aid of the pineal gland (*Scientific American,* 1965).

neal gland of cattle responsible for the pallidness of embryonal amphibian skin. The compound proved to be an indole derivative and was given the name of *melatonin.*

Evolutionary History of the Pineal Gland

Studies have shown that an organ was formed at the beginning of the evolution of living creatures with the function of transmitting heat and light as well as vibrations of the air to the body to stimulate reactions to danger, to reproduce, and so on. This organ, which later developed into the pineal gland, may be considered the original form taken by our sensory organs. Even in the case of invertebrates (e.g., crabs and insects) there is, in addition to the two facet eyes, a structure ("the parietal eye of insects") corresponding to the pineal organ of vertebrates. This apparently developed before the two laterally situated eyes. Among the oldest

animals on the evolutionary scale we find the jawless fish (lamprey). Up until the time of its metamorphosis into the sexually mature animal, the hatched larva of the lamprey has only the medial pineal eye; the rudiments of the lateral eyes do not develop until after metamorphosis.

In the course of phylogenesis, the pineal organ becomes a tubular structure, one end of which forms the vesicular, protuberant pineal eye while the other connects with the cerebrospinal system. A histological make-up is found similar to that of sensory organs. In the case of later-evolving amphibians, typical sensory cells can be detected by means of the electron microscope. Reptiles (e.g., sauria, lizards, snakes, turtles) show the highest development of the pineal gland as a sensory organ. In their case it has an incomplete ocular structure that contains a miniature cornea, lens, and conical retina with nerve fibers emanating from it. This organ protrudes from the skull of lizards, looking like an eye covered with skin. After having first been described as a thermoregulatory organ (von Frisch), it was then assumed to be a transmitter of environmental light and color stimuli to the organism, although itself being incapable of visual perception. Among reptiles, however, there are species which do not display any typical sensory cells in their pineal organ (e.g., iguana, ring snake). In certain species, a reduction in thickness of the cellular layer of the pineal organ and its transition to a gland-like form may be observed.

In birds, the pineal organ, which had formerly been a sensory organ, is totally converted into a gland which betrays traces of its history only in the embryonic stage. Sensory receptors begin forming in the pineal organ of 14- to 18-day-old chicken embryos. This development ceases two days after hatching. The birds have a pineal gland which is saccular, vesicular, or—as in mammals—compact.

When this morphological transformation of the pineal gland occurs in more highly evolved animals it is accompanied simultaneously by a functional change from sensory organ to endocrine gland. The mammalian pineal gland, for example, no longer has any sensory functions; it has become a ductless gland. But even in the case of mammals the pineal gland retains its functional connection with light, one of its former basic characteristics. In mammals, photostimulus is no longer transmitted as it is in the lower vertebrates by the pineal vesicle that is located directly under the skull. It is now the eyes that relay the effect of light to the pineal gland by way of the sympathetic nervous system.

Melatonin

Neural impulses induced by light in turn stimulate the pineal gland to secrete a hormone, melatonin, which—once released into the bloodstream—travels to and affects the gonads and the pituitary, adrenal, and thyroid glands. This hormone was discovered when the sexual maturation of rats was inhibited by injections with pineal extracts. By fractionation and purification of the pineal extract, melatonin was isolated and demonstrated to be the active inhibiting substance. In mammals it is believed to be produced in the pinealocytes which develop from the embryonic neural epithelium. Melatonin, the specific hormone of the pineal gland, has also been discovered in humans.

By contracting the pigmentary granules of the melanocytes, melatonin causes pallidness in fish, reptiles, and amphibians, thus counteracting the hormone (chromatophore hormone) that stimulates melanocytes and is synthesized in the intermediate region of the pituitary gland.

Light and Darkness

Experiments with animals in constant light and constant darkness established the fact that the synthesis of melatonin is governed by light. The synthesis of melatonin from serotonin (N-acetylserotonin) (preliminary stage: tryptophane) is catalyzed by HIOMT which is present in high concentrations exclusively in the pineal gland of mammals (Axelrod et al 1964). Light apparently inhibits this enzyme in nocturnal animals, whereas darkness performs the same function in diurnal ones. Furthermore, not only melatonin synthesis but also excretion is increased in darkness in both humans and experimental animals (Lynch et al 1975).

Constant light (6 to 55 days) leads to diminished activity of HIOMT in the rat and consequently to a reduction in the melatonin production of the pineal gland. Constant darkness increases the activity so that more melatonin is produced. This effect of light on HIOMT appears to be specific since the activity of other enzymes present in the pineal gland is not influenced by light. Possibly the influence of light on HIOMT occurs by means of secretion of noradrenalin, for an increase of this hormone inhibits the enzyme.

Another enzyme—the pineal gland's N-acetyltransferase—also appears to play a key role in the synthesis of melatonin. It signals vertebrates as to whether it is day or night, regardless of whether the animal in question is diurnal or nocturnal.

The Influence of Light via Retina–Pineal Gland

The question now arises as to how light influences the production of melatonin in the pineal gland. There is no doubt that neural pathways exist between the retina and the hypothalamus. The experimental employment of photostimuli and of darkness, as well as metabolic studies of the blind as compared with those with normal sight, furnish unequivocal proof of this. Moreover, light-evoked potentials can be traced in the hypothalamus of rats. In the rat, enucleation of the eye and lesion in the areas of the accessory optic nerve bundle and the sympathetic nervous system interrupt the effect of photostimuli on the pineal gland. Severing the optic tract behind the optic chiasm, on the other hand, does not influence light's effect on the pineal gland.

From an anatomical point of view, it is possible for light to influence the pineal gland in the following ways:

1) Light penetrates the skull, affecting the pineal gland directly by activating photoreceptive elements. This possibility exists only for lower animals; up to the present, no characteristic photoreceptors have been found in the pineal gland of mammals. It has been proved that light ceases to affect the pineal gland of adult rats after enucleation of both eyes. It must therefore be assumed that light's effect on mammals takes place by means of retinal photoreceptors in the eyes and not by means of the direct effect of light on the pineal gland.

2) Light influences the pineal gland by means of other neuroendocrine transmitting materials, i.e., pituitary hormones. Hypophysectomized rats continued to demonstrate the stimulating effect of light on the production of melatonin by the pineal gland so that the possibility of a pituitary transmitter can be dismissed. Although there are proven interactions between the pituitary and pineal gland, the pituitary does not appear to play an essential role in transferring the effect of photostimuli to the pineal gland.

3) By way of the hypothalamus and the pituitary gland, light influences sexual maturation without the intervention of the pineal gland. Numerous authors have demonstrated the existence of direct neural pathways leading from the retina to the hypothalamus. Others, in turn, have cast doubt on these findings. Autoradiographic methods recently applied to guinea pigs, rats, cats, and monkeys have shown direct connections between the retina and the hypothalamus ending in the supraoptic nucleus of the hypothalamus but in no other region of that organ (Moore and Lenn 1972; Hendrickson et al 1972; Meier 1973).

4) Another possible way for light to influence the pineal gland is by means of the autonomic nervous system. Sympathetic nerve fibers leading from the superior cervical ganglion to the pineal gland were discovered in rats (Kappers 1960). Severing the individual nerve fibers in the rat disclosed pathways which conduct photostimuli from the retina to the sympathetic nervous system (see Fig. 11).

Examinations conducted after exstirpation of the superior cervical ganglion and after severing the sympathetic nerve fibers lead to the conclusion that photostimuli reach the pineal gland by this pathway.

The pineal gland functions as a neuroendocrine transmitter by transforming neural stimuli into hormonal ones (melatonin) under the influence of an exogenous factor (light); these hormonal stimuli then reach the midbrain and pituitary gland (and thereby the gonads) through the bloodstream (Wurtman and Weisel 1969).

Melatonin inhibits gonad function principally by modifying the secretion of gonadotropic hormones in the anterior lobe of the pituitary gland. Changes in the adenohypophysis have been demonstrated after pinealectomy. After a certain time, alterations in the function of the pineal gland no longer affect the gonads (Sayler and Wolfson 1968), i.e., normal sexual activity is ultimately possible even without the pineal gland (Kappers 1969). What is involved here then is a modifying influence of the pineal gland or, in other words, one part of a finely demarcated regulatory system in the hypothalamus.

It should be noted that these experiments were carried out principally on rats, which are nocturnal. The pineal gland of birds, which are diurnal, behaves in an opposite fashion; in this case, the synthesis of melatonin is stimulated, not inhibited, by light (Axelrod et al 1964). Recent experiments showed that melatonin may be involved in mediating a photoperiod response in hamsters (Tamarkin and Goldman 1977). From experimental studies (Wolfson and Turek 1977) of the photosensitive white-throated sparrow—unlike their results in the hamster—melatonin does not appear to play a role in the photoperiodic regulation of the avian gonadal cycle.

Interaction of the Pineal with Other Endocrine Glands

There have been numerous descriptions of the pineal gland's interactions with other endocrine glands, especially the pituitary. Various stimuli influence the pituitary and pineal glands in opposite ways. These two organs are almost always related in their regulation of peripheral endocrine glands, the pituitary exercising a positive stimulatory effect, the pineal a negative inhibitory one (Kühnau 1971).

Receptor organs of the pineal's hormonal secretion are essentially the gonads, the thyroid, and the adrenal gland.

Effect on the Gonads

Experiments with animals and clinical observations indicate that a hypofunction of the pineal leads to pubertas praecox (see the section on blind children) and a hyperfunction to a delayed appearance of puberty.

The pineal gland inhibits the secretion of the gonadotropic hormone by the anterior lobe of the pituitary. Recent experimental work indicates that there is, in addition to this direct influence on the pituitary, also an indirect one through the mediation of the hypothalamus. Very recently, Vaughan, Meyer, and Reiter (1978) published a review about the evidence of a pineal–gonad relationship in humans.

Effect on the Thyroid Gland

Pineal extracts diminish the activity of the thyroid gland by inhibiting the pituitary thyrotropic hormone. Pinealectomy causes thyroid hyperfunction. Here too, therefore, an inhibitory influence is apparent.

Effect on the Adrenal Cortex

It is assumed today that the pineal gland can actively produce an aldosterone secretion, i.e., under physiological conditions it par-

takes in the mechanism of reabsorption of water and salt. Testing of these assumptions is still in its initial stages.

In summary, the observations and experiments made to date clearly indicate that the pineal gland is a center of neuroendocrine regulation which converts photostimuli as well as impulses stemming from the autonomic nervous system into hormonal messages (Wurtman, Axelrod et al 1963, 1964a,b, 1968).

Light and Color Change

Lister performed the first experiments involving blinded frogs in 1885. He was able to show that an animal which has adapted to darkness no longer demonstrates any color change after enucleation: it stays a dark color in bright light. The effect of light of various wave lengths on color change in amphibians was also described in the last century. In 1886 Hermann discovered that salamander larvae grow lighter when exposed to red light and darker when exposed to blue light.

Stutinsky (1939) established the fact that the eyeless frog assumes a permanent intermediate coloration which remains constant regardless of the degree of brightness of the environment. Rodewald (1935) covered the frog's eyes with a light-proof cap. When Hollwich (1958) sutured the frog's lids, color change came to a halt and the frog assumed an intermediate shade of color (see Fig. 5). Both observations attest to the importance of the eyes' reception of photostimuli and the subsequent transmission of these stimuli to the pituitary gland.

As mentioned in the introductory remarks, Mast (1916) was able to prove that color change in the plaice proceeds via the eye.

In the photometric measurement of color change in the plaice and sole, Wilhelm (1969) found that the extent of pigment concentration at the range of 1–4,000 lux depends on the logarithm of the light intensity. In the case of series of stimuli, summation—or facilitation and adaptation—was observed to depend on the duration of the intervals.

There were also early suggestions that the pituitary gland was involved in color change in amphibians. Allen (1917) showed that frogs turned permanently pale after extirpation of the pituitary.

Hogben (1922, 1924) was then able to prove that pallescense in the frog after extirpation of the pituitary originates from a deficiency of the pituitary hormone. The animals thus operated on turned dark again after being injected with vertebrate pituitary extract.

It was Jores (1935, 1938) who confirmed that the melanophore hormone is of essential importance for man as well as for animals. He found pronounced, diurnally periodic fluctuations which were dependent on the light-darkness alternation in the level of melanophore hormones in the blood and in the pituitary gland.

In 1958, Hollwich, by making the frog's visual center inoperative by means of coagulation, succeeded in proving that color change occurs independently of the visual process (see Figs. 8C and 8D). Via the eye and an "energetic portion" of the visual pathway distinguishable from the "optic portion," photostimuli reach the diencephalon, where they influence the pituitary gland's hormone production.

4

Light and Growth

Size and weight are the most important measurements for assessing body development. It must not be forgotten, however, that physiologically both of these vary considerably, and that heredity, standard of living, and the acceleration of growth which can be measured from generation to generation play a large role. Aside from these factors, body growth and development evince a series of features more or less clearly connected with the manner in which the endocrine glands function and thus with the production of hormones.

Height and weight, as well as the area of the body's surface, the musculature, the skeleton, and other organs usually exhibit a relatively uniform growth. More exact analysis discloses four different periods: First, the body grows extraordinarily quickly. Then, until puberty, there follows a slower but relatively constant growth which runs approximately parallel to the weight curve of the pituitary and thyroid glands. Puberty is accompanied by a renewed spurt of growth obviously connected with the sudden increase in weight of the gonads and adrenal glands and their production of sex hormones. The puberal spurt in growth gradually subsides until growth comes to a complete halt.

The Influence of Light on the Growth and Development of Invertebrates

The direct influence of light on the growth and development of invertebrates was demonstrated by Belyaeva (1939). If silkworm colonies are exposed to continuous artificial illumination during the night hours, the production of finished silk increases by 6.5 percent and the average weight of the cocoon by 5.8 percent. Shortening the daily period of illumination to only 12 hours brought about a decrease in silk production of 5.8 percent.

On the basis of experiments with the corn beetle, V. Törne (1941) proved that the intensity and color of light have an influence on development and reproduction. Red light and total darkness turned out to be especially unfavorable in this connection, whereas yellow and moderately subdued light had a stimulating effect.

The development of butterflies from caterpillars likewise appears to depend upon illumination. Müller (1955, 1956) raised caterpillars under thoroughly uniform conditions, with the exception that at one time they were subjected to long day conditions (16 hours of light), at another to short day conditions (8 hours of light). Under long day conditions an acceleration of development ensued.

The influence of the amount of environmental light on appetite, weight, and growth in length of a certain species of lizard was described by Fox and Dessauer (1957). Their work does not make clear, however, whether ocularly perceived light was the determining factor.

Bünning and Joerrens (1960) came to similar conclusions about the development of the cabbage butterfly: short day conditions induced a diapause (a phase of rest in the development of insects), whereas this was inhibited in the case of the long day.

Williams (1963) was able to prove that the light penetrating the cocoon works directly on the brain. Stimulation of the neurosecretory cells causes the secretion of a cerebral hormone responsible for the further development of the pupa.

The Influence of Light on the Development of the Human Body and Mind

Experimental evidence on light's influence on human body and mental development results from studies demonstrating the effect of the lack of perceived light by the blind. Today's attentive observer is not the first to note the influence of blindness in childhood on the development of the human body and mind. Wimmer (1856) writes about the inmates of Munich's Royal Institution for the Blind:

> Just as the color, shape, taste, and smell of plants are altered by a lack of light, so, when eyesight is extinguished, vegetative life continues as imperfectly as if the human being were

in a dark place where he was deprived of the influence of light, that all-enlivening element; for the eyes are the transmitters of light for the organism.

And in another passage:

> The whole appearance of a blind person when deprived of sight for a long period of time bears the markings of that underdeveloped vegetative state, of that retarded growth due to deficient bone formation, poor mixture of vital fluids, and the pallor thus caused—all of which make the body disposed to diseases difficult to cure, especially to rachitic deformities and to scrofulous diseases. But this underdeveloped vegetative state disappears again, the body's power of reproduction is enlivened anew, and the organism seems to grow younger when vision is restored—for example by a cataract operation or the formation of an artificial pupil—to someone who has been blind for a long period.

In 1927 the orthopedist Lange examined the children at the Munich Institution for the Blind, finding frequent deformities of the torso such as otherwise occur only rarely (Fig. 13). This was true, however, only for children who had been blind since birth. When a child did not become blind until his eighth, tenth, or 14th year, it generally displayed the same posture as most other schoolchildren. The author attributed the cause of the deformities of the torso, the retarded growth, and the skeletal problems to early blindness, lack of physical exercise, and lack of light.

Yano (1954) evaluated the Ministry of Education's statistics which recorded the height and weight of all school children. He came to the conclusion that blind children up to the age of five or six do not differ in height from those with normal vision of the same age. Later, however, the average increase in growth clearly rises more sharply in normal children, reaching a maximal difference at the age of 18 to 19. The standard deviation from the average values for height is substantially greater in blind children; they exhibit a substantially more irregular growth increase than their peers with normal vision. It seemed noteworthy, in addition, that blind

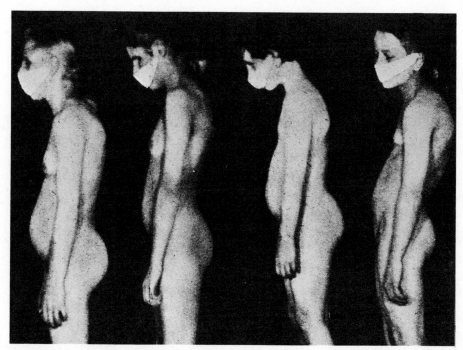

Fig. 13.   According to Lange (1927), those who become blind early in life exhibit retarded growth and abnormal skeletal development.

girls were ahead of blind boys in growth for a longer period than usual.

Saller (1961) also reports on variations in height of 58 male and 55 female inmates of the Bavarian Institute for the Blind. In the case of this sample, which was not homogeneous as to the time blindness occurred, he found that growth proceeds regularly as far as increase in height is concerned but that it is clearly retarded in all age groups. He ascribes this growth deficiency in the blind to the lack of photostimulus, among other factors: "heliogenic acceleration via retina and pituitary."

On the basis of observations of 694 blind children in Karl Marx-Stadt, Liebe and Keller (1965) found that blind children are more frequently retarded than children with normal vision in regard to speed of growth and to intellectual development. Those who became blind early (in the first year of life) were considerably more affected than those who became blind later (after the first year). The authors leave open the question as to the ultimate cause of the retardation, since

in their opinion the general lack of contact and an injury causing the blindness could also be involved along with the failure of light to strike the retina.

Using the Vogt somatogram, Kaloud (1970) studied growth in blind children. Compared with normal children of the same age, their bodies are clearly underdeveloped. There are differences in the case of amaurotic patients insofar as blind children show the strongest deviations beginning at birth, with only a slight increase in growth occurring after their 12th year. Those regaining their sight by means of surgery exhibit a spurt in growth, and children becoming blind late (after puberty) show no difference from those with normal vision.

We observed that blind girls reach their menarche half to one year earlier compared with sighted girls. This is a remarkable difference between the retarded development of growth and the earlier sexual maturation of blind girls. Wurtman, Axelrod, and Phillips (1963), Zacharias and Wurtman (1964), Wurtman and Weisel (1969), and Axelrod

(1970) found the pineal hormone melatonin likely to be the substance that caused gonad inhibition. Therefore, light input via the eyes stimulates and its absence diminishes the formation of a gonad-inhibiting substance in the pineal.

Sella–Pituitary Growth

An explanation for the retarded growth and much smaller increase in the height of children who became blind early in life is offered by the data on sellar area presented by Hollwich in 1951. X-ray examinations of the skull indicated that the blind have a sella which is smaller in area on the average than that of persons with sight. Conspicuous here was the fact that it is predominantly those becoming blind early in life who possess smaller than normal sellae. On the other hand, the sellar areas of those who became blind later in life lie within the range of the norm (Fig. 14).

An explanation for this condition is given by the developmental curve of the normal sella. This is divided into two stages: in the first five years of life the sella attains 80 percent of its surface area in rapid growth; during the following 15 years it grows the remaining 20 percent gradually.

In accord with these findings, the analysis of the sellar area of 74 blind persons showed that the time at which blindness occurred influences the development of the sella. If it occurred in the first years of life, the sella usually remains small. If it occurs later, i.e., in the second developmental stage, then larger sellar areas result. Since the pituitary is located in the intrasellar area, very small sellae also mean smaller, i.e., hypoplastic, pituitaries. This leads to the conclusion that photostimuli also have a stimulatory effect on the development of the pituitary. These experiments were corroborated by Fuchs (1953), von Schumann (1953), Büchner and Kukla (1954), as well as by Wassner (1954).

The Growth Hormone (HGH)

The growth of an organism depends on orderly metabolic functioning and sufficient nourishment, but the actual impulse for

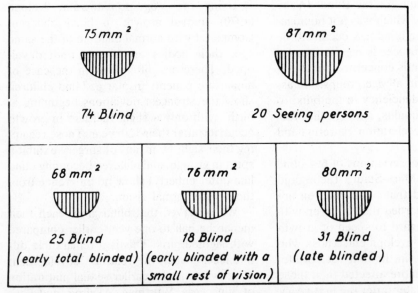

Fig. 14.   Schematic graph of the average value of the sella plane of 74 blind and 20 normal control persons (scale 1:1).

growth proceeds from the growth hormone. The human growth hormone *(HGH)** plays a role in a large number of vital processes. The *anabolic* effect is manifested in nitrogen retention, the increased transport of amino acids to the cell, increased synthesis of protein accompanying the formation of *DNA*† and ribosomes, and also in its influence on the activity of bone marrow and of cellular defense. The anabolic effect is paralleled by a *catabolic* effect: gluconeogenesis from proteins is decreased by mobilizing energy from fat deposits in case energy needs are not being met continuously. As an insulin antagonist HGH inhibits glucose utilization, especially in the musculature, and thereby raises the level of blood sugar. More insulin is needed to bring glucose to the cells. The diabetogenic effect, earlier described as the "contra-insular principle of the pituitary," also explains the heightened insulin sensitivity of an organism after hypophysectomy. In this connection attention should be called to our experiments with those becoming blind when young who suffered from pituitary hypofunction and who reacted to an insulin tolerance test with a drop in blood sugar (see p. 63).

The effect of the growth hormone on water balance is partly a renotropic one consisting of an increase in tubular secretion and electrolyte retention. The increase in skin turgor is to be ascribed more to the increased synthesis of water-retaining extracellular substances. These functions of the hormone are naturally essential not only during the age of growth but also after full body height is attained since protein utilization continues throughout life. Another name for HGH—the somatotropic hormone—indicates this situation. The growth-fostering effect of the hormone appears to be constituted of several specific effects. Along with the anabolic effects influencing the entire organism, a protein that acts specifically upon bone growth originates under the influence of this hormone: it is called the "sulfation factor," also known today as somatomedin. Normal growth results only when all factors work together harmoniously (Butenandt 1974).

Since it has become possible to analyze the growth hormone with radioimmunological methods, many authors have recently turned their attention to the clarification of the circadian rhythm of HGH. Kowarski et al (1971) described a portable pump for the extended collection of blood in order to analyze the course of this hormone's secretion. De Laet et al (1974) attempted to demonstrate by these same means a daily curve for the growth hormone. The fluctuations in HGH plasma level were so slight, however, that it was possible to establish in merely summary fashion that there was a higher secretion of HGH during the period from 6 P.M. to 6 A.M. than from 6 A.M. to 6 P.M. By the additional application of radioactively marked HGH, Alford et al (1973) were able to trace the hormone's metabolization. They discovered that the secretion of the growth hormone was almost three times greater at night than during the day. The change from a lying to an upright position had a strong influence on the rate of metabolization. Plotnik et al (1975) traced HGH's circadian rhythm in children, teenagers, and young adults under conditions of normal physical activity. In all three groups, during the day as well as at night during sleep, peaks of secretory activity occurred. These were lower, however, for the adults than for the children and teenagers. Plasma levels, low during the early morning hours, showed a steady rise until evening. Food intake did not cause any significant changes. During the night the growth hormone level again fell back to the low morning values. Since the half-life period of HGH—determined from the fall in plasma level—was significantly higher than the true half-life period of metabolization, the authors concluded that at no

*Peptide hormone of the pituitary gland; influences growth, fat and glucose metabolism (diabetogenic effect). Newer desigation is somatotropic hormone (STH).

†Deoxyribonucleic acid: characteristic component of nucleic proteins.

time of day is there complete inactivity in HGH secretion such as is postulated, for example, for adrenocorticotropic hormone (ACTH).*

Hollwich (1973) and Dieckhues (1974) presented the first data on the influence of ocular light perception on the HGH level. There is not only a significant difference in HGH level between the seeing and the blind, but in the case of a cataract patient a significant rise in the level can be determined after removal of the cataract and complete restitution of light's entry into the eye. On the other hand, there is no difference between the blind and the seeing in the level of hydroxyproline as parameter for the formation of collagen. If the daily curves of HGH secretion in the seeing and the blind are compared with each other (Dieckhues 1974), it is striking, first, that the daily fluctuations (amplitudes) are lower, and, second, that the mean daily figures are lower for the blind than for those with normal vision. This research demonstrates again that the function of the organism is very closely connected with daylight and the alternation between light and dark. When light is cut off completely, as, for example, in the case of blindness, its stimulatory and regulatory effect is absent, the diurnal rhythmic fluctuations are barely discernible any longer, hormone secretion is severely diminished, and there is a "neuroendocrine deficit." It would appear that the individual hormonal regulatory systems are still intact but that their normal activity is reduced.

*Regulates glucocorticoid synthesis (cortisol, cortisone, androgen) in the zona fasciculata and reticularis of the adrenal cortex.

5

Light and Body Temperature

When we speak about human body temperature, it must be understood that all parts of the body do not have the same temperature. Rather, there exists a complicated spatial temperature field which is also subject to temporal variations. The heat produced inside the organism is constantly flowing outward; thus, for purely physical reasons a temperature variance occurs between the internal and external parts of the body. In addition, there is a temperature drop in the extremities from proximal to distal so that an axial as well as a radial temperature variance exists.

It is important to distinguish a homoiothermal (warm blooded) body core from a poikilothermal (of varying temperature) body surface. The interior of the torso and of the head constitute the body core, the skin and extremities constitute the body surface. External and internal influences on body temperature (air temperature and movement, atmospheric humidity, physical labor) call for an equalization in temperature. Essential for the regulation of heat emission (physical thermoregulation) is the transfer of heat to the body surface through the circulation of the blood. From there, heat emission

ensues by means of radiation, convection, conduction, and evaporation—depending on the organism's function and activity in its different parts. Heat production (chemical thermoregulation) ensues as a result both of metabolism of the liver and other internal organs and of the release of mechanical and chemical energy in the skeletal muscle. The hypothalamic region in particular is of decisive importance in the regulation of temperature. The thermoregulatory centers react to local changes in temperature and perform the function of temperature antennae that are influenced directly by the core temperature and indirectly by skin temperature. Impulses reach the heat center by reflection via the skin's thermoreceptors, the temperature of the blood itself, and the direct influence of heat or cold on the cutaneous vessels. Thermoregulation is maintained with the aid of positive and negative feedback mechanisms.

Diurnal Rhythm of Body Temperature in Adults

The first studies concerning body temperature changes throughout the day were done by Jürgensen (1873). According to his investigations, maximum temperature occurs between 5 P.M. and 8 P.M., minimum temperature between 2 A.M. and 6 A.M. Jürgensen found the average difference between minimum and maximum to be one degree Centigrade. Liebermeister (1875) soon established that this temperature change is essentially independent of external factors such as activity, diet, and sleep.

By means of maximum elimination of muscular activity, Johannson (1898) obtained a substantial reduction in, but not a complete elimination of, the daily fluctuations in temperature. On the basis of this, he concluded that the cause of the diurnal–nocturnal rhythm was to be found in the physical work and exercise associated with the day and the rest associated with the night.

According to Hörmann (1898), nocturnal rest as well as lack of food intake causes a drop in temperature. He explained the absence of temperature fluctuations in a stuporous patient as the result of elimination of external stimuli, especially light.

According to Völker (1927), a change in living habits—not only in the form of a direct reversal but also a shift in schedule of six to eight hours—is probably capable of shifting the temperature rhythm but not eliminating it completely. In making a comparison with temperature curves done in Iceland, he ascertained that there is a local time link with the sun, although it does not have any further influence. Völker sees the rhythms of the life processes he studied as "subject to an as yet undetermined cosmic principle."

Forsgren (1929, 1935) sees the 24-hour variation in body temperature along with fluid excretion as determined predominantly by liver function, although he is unable to explain the cause. Menzel (1950) also reports on a characteristic body rhythm whereby the temperature curve coincides with the diuresis curve. Menzel (1962) reports on changes in axillary temperature (or body surface temperature) during the winter season. The maximum in winter is said to be at 3 P.M., in summer at 8 P.M.

Diurnal Rhythm of Body Temperature in Infants

The development of periodic diurnal temperature regulation shows itself very clearly in the infant in the course of the first weeks and months of life. The first extensive investigations in this area were done by Jundell (1904). He attributes the observable increase in temperature amplitudes in the course of development to the decrease in temperature during the night.

Mullin (1939) reports that the temperature curve is established with regularity from the sixth month on and is fully developed from the eleventh month on. He confirms that amplitude owes its initial increase to the drop in night temperatures. Kleitman et al (1937) observed that daily temperature fluctuations start increasing virtually from birth. This early development of periodicity from the fifth day of life on had already been mentioned by von Bärensprung (1851) and more precisely described and explained by Sommer (1880). The curves done by de Rudder and Petersen (1935) were based on the temperatures of one- to three-month-old infants; an amplitude of .45 degree Centigrade was found. The extremely extensive and careful measurements and records made by Kleitman and Engelmann (1953) confirm that a clear-cut sleep–waking periodicity is already established in the infant in the first four weeks of life.

Hellbrügge (1965) also later analyzed Jundell's data and enlarged upon them through his own observations of schoolchildren. In the first to third weeks of life body temperatures do not exhibit any day–night difference. The daytime level does not rise until the fifth to tenth week. However, the infants do not show a clear indication of day–night periodicity until the tenth to sixteenth week, at which time there is an increase in the daytime figures and also a decrease in the nighttime temperature. Especially in the case of the development of sleep periodicity in infants—studied extensively by Kleitman and Engelmann (1953) and Parmelee (1961)—Hellbrügge speaks of the infant's innate circadian periodicity, based on an endogenic self-induced oscillation. In the course of the first weeks of life, depending on the degree of maturation of the organ or system in question, it gradually changes into a 24-hour periodicity.

Disturbances in Temperature Rhythm Caused by Changes in Diurnal Rhythm

Numerous studies have been conducted on the reaction of body temperature when the normal 24-hour activity rhythm is changed. By means of electric registration of temperature, Benedict and Snell (1902) monitored the rectal temperature of a night worker. For 12 nights they took a reading every four minutes and on the last day during the day as well. In spite of certain irregularities the studies clearly show that the basic outline of the temperature curve is in no way influenced by the reversal of life pattern. Benedict (1904–1905) repeated the experiments with a night watchman who had been following a reversed life pattern for eight years without interruption, finding the same result: there was no sign of any adaptation to this reversed sleep–waking rhythm.

As early as 1927 Völker pointed out that reversal of life pattern, while producing no direct reverse in temperature rhythms, nevertheless is probably capable of causing it to shift. Bjerner and Swensson (1954) characterize the specific quality of shift work as it influences diurnal rhythm. The shift worker does have the possibility of acting in opposition to his environment's periodicity but remains conscious of this unusual action and as a result retains a connection with the original periodicity and its time indicators (clocks). Hildebrandt's (1973) opinion on the reversal of life pattern is that in shift work only a few functions are able to adapt themselves to this reversal. He found that body temperature continues to reach a maximum during the day and a minimum during the night. The change from light to darkness by itself does not suffice to in-

vert all of man's biologic functions as it does in the case of animals.

Experiments with isolation can also be informative about the nature time indicators must have if an individual who has been cut off from his environment is to retain his circadian periodicity. In Kleitman's cave experiment (1939) the body temperature of his co-worker assumed a new rhythm after a sleep–waking rhythm of 28 hours which had lasted for several weeks. In the case of Kleitman himself, the 24-hour body temperature rhythm remained constant. Menzel (1962) brought about total inversion in body temperature of a 27-year-old bed-ridden microcephalic patient by changing the lighting and the pattern of food intake.

Mills and Stanbury (1952) found in the case of five experimental subjects kept in a basement that even with an artificial sleep-waking rhythm of 12 hours the 24-hour body temperature rhythm remained constant.

The research group Aschoff, Pöppel, and Wever (1969) conducted experiments for three to four weeks in complete isolation, with free choice regarding daily schedule and lighting. Under these conditions a shift of 12 hours appeared by the 12th day in the measurement of body functions (body temperature, beginning of activity, and maximum urinary excretion), including the sleep-waking rhythm. The mean diurnal period was lengthened by one hour and amounted to 25.9 hours. With a change in the experimental conditions, i.e., a transition from weak to brighter lighting, the three measured functions decreased by .6 to 1.0 hours. In a second experiment with reversed sequence, i.e., a transition from brighter to weaker lighting, periodicity was increased by an equal amount.

Wever (1969) discusses the hypothesis that by closing the eyes a light–darkness alternation continues to exist, even with constant lighting. The same conditions would then exist as with optional lighting. But as experience shows, merely closing the eyelids is not sufficient to eliminate fully the perception of light. The use of eye covers during naps proves this. In a room illuminated by artificial or natural light, anyone can prove for himself that light also penetrates closed eyelids. Perception of light is completely eliminated only when we hold both hands over our closed eyes.

The influence of perception of even slight amounts of light is confirmed by studies (to be cited later) of temperature reactions (Jores 1934a,b, 1935a) and metabolism (Hollwich 1948–1974) in the case of complete or partial absence of light perception.

Further experiments by the above-mentioned research group of Aschoff, Pöppel, and Wever (1969) indicate that an artificial light-darkness alternation adjusts human circadian periodicity only to periods of approximately 24 hours. Thus, when all time indicators have been eliminated, an endogenic independent periodicity may exist.

Interruptions in Temperature Rhythm in the Blind

As early as 1934 Jores observed four virtually blind persons during a one-day con-finement to darkness. In two cases he noted a suspension of temperature rhythm and in the other two a distinctly altered rhythm. He concluded that even in the case of the blind, light is one factor among others to which we must ascribe an influence on the 24-hour periodicity of temperature regulation. Remler (1948), unlike Jores, does not believe that the light-darkness alternation influences human diurnal periodicity.

In their water immersion test, Tromp and Bouma (1967) established without question that 41 blind boys ranging in age from 6 to 18 had an insufficient thermoregulatory mechanism.

In summary, we can say that human body temperature reaches a high point in the course of the day and during the night sinks to a low point: This temperature rhythm, however, is subject to slight individual variations. When all exterior "time indicators" are experimentally eliminated, independent periods of individual body functions appear which differ in length and can be modified by numerous external influences. In this connection, temperature rhythm is a relatively constant factor.

6
Light and Kidney Function

Observations concerning the temporal aspects of water excretion go back to the last century. The first exhaustive studies, which are still relevant today, were made by Quincke (1877, 1893). Quincke was the first to observe the matutinal flow of urine. From this observation as well as from experiments demonstrating that the nocturnal decrease in urine occurs only when sleeping in a horizontal position, Quincke concludes that this position promotes excretion of urine. Jores (1935) conducted tests pertaining to this question on ten night watchmen. He divided fluid intake equally over a period of 24 hours, with food intake occurring only during the night. The relationship between diurnal and nocturnal urine patterns did not change. A further shift toward diurnal excretion even became evident. A recumbent position during the day promoted water excretion, as already discovered by Quincke and, after him, a whole series of investigators (Seyderhelm and Goldberg 1927). Jores concludes from this that sleep as such cannot directly inhibit water excretion, especially since among his experimental subjects there was one person who had been continuously

employed for eight years as a night watchman so that the deficiency of excretion during the experiment could not be the result of adaptation to the reversal in life pattern.

Besides sleep, it has been above all the lack of fluid and food intake which, since Quincke's time, has been seen as the cause of this condition. There are numerous studies along these lines, for example, one by Campbell and Webster (1922), who had their subjects go without food and liquid during the day and let them eat and drink at night, and those by Simpson (1924, 1926) and Jores (1935), who administered fluids every two hours to their subjects. All these experiments indicated that there was no variation in the temporal aspects of water excretion.

Forsgren (1935) connected the rhythmic variations in kidney function with liver function; the secretory, i.e., disassimilatory, phase of metabolic activity is followed by increased diuresis, i.e., by a "flow of water and disassimilation products," along with an increase in heat production and body temperature. Simultaneously with the assimilatory phase, diuresis tapers off and body temperature drops. Forsgren sees the rhythmic function of the kidneys in the total context of the body's metabolism and rejects an independent rhythm of diuresis.

By administering equal amounts of water every hour to two experimental groups consisting of 42 and 35 subjects respectively, Gerritzen (1938) was able to demonstrate that the 24-hour rhythm of diuresis reaches a minimum after midnight and a maximum around 1 P.M.. Since the alimentary intake was the same every hour and diuresis exhibited a distinct rhythm, the kidney's rhythmic impulse must originate in the organism itself, i.e., in the liver, according to Gerritzen's view.

Menzel (1950) studied the diurnal rhythm of both urine excretion and rectal temperature in the case of 26 ill and healthy people confined to bed. Over a 24-hour period the amount of urine as well as the urine's chloride, urea, and creatinine content along with the rectal temperature were measured every three hours. According to Menzel's conclusions, kidney function customarily occurs in a 24-hour rhythm and in integral segments of 24 hours.

Sirota et al (1950) studied diurnal fluctuations in kidney function in 18 healthy males to whom they administered test substances continuously (inulin and para amino hippuric acid [PAH]) normally found in the urine. The day–night relationship of urine flow, measured by means of both test substances, showed a significant decrease in urine flow at night along with an increase in tubular water reabsorption and a relatively constant glomerular rate of filtration and plasma flow. Corresponding to the deep sleep phase from midnight to 4 A.M., the glomerular filtration rate also declines. Thus, the decrease in urine production is attributed mainly to an increased nocturnal rate of water reabsorption.

Water Balance

On a wall relief in Egypt, Fuchs (1965) discovered a blind harpist with a puffy face and bloated habitus, in other words, with signs of a disturbed water balance. If the inducing influence of light is lacking—as is the case with the blind—a modification of water balance occurs (Hollwich 1948). For someone with sight, normal diuresis is distinguished by a small amount of urine excreted nocturnally with a high specific gravity and by a larger amount excreted during the day with a low specific gravity. The modification of water balance in the blind person causes us to conclude that he experiences reduced efficiency of the antidiuretic pituitary hormone which is normally active at night. This becomes especially apparent when the water balance is subjected to stress by Volhard's water loading test or when, in addition, the antidiuretic hormone of the posterior pituitary lobe is injected. Tests of 67 blind persons compared to 20 persons with normal sight revealed that the blind have a lesser amount of diurnal urine whereas the amount excreted nocturnally increases in the form of nocturia (Fig. 15). The totally blind therefore very often display a puffy appearance and bloated habitus (Fig. 16).

In order to eliminate exogenic factors, Hollwich (1955; Hollwich and Dieckhues 1974a,b) also performed the Volhard water

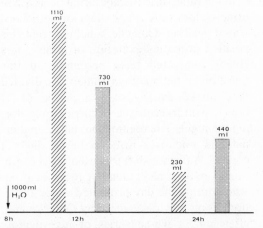

Fig. 15. The Volhard water balance test on the blind in comparison with the normal sighted. The four-hour water excretion is lower in the blind than in the normal sighted, whereas nocturnal water excretion in the blind increases compared to the normal sighted (nocturia). Hatched bar, sighted (n = 20); shaded bar, blind (n = 67).

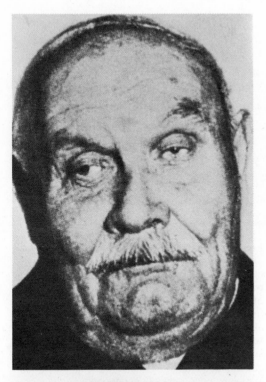

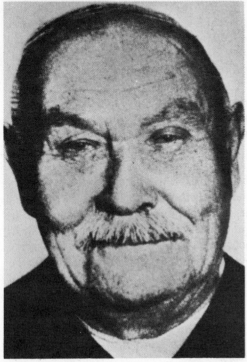

test on patients who for all practical purposes had been blind for years as a result of cataracts of *both* eyes (Fig. 17). Just as in the previous case of the blind, the amount of urine was also less during the day whereas nocturnal excretion was increased in the form of nocturia. Postoperatively—after removal of the cataracts and restoration of light's entry into the eye (Fig. 17)—the Volhard water test on these same patients showed normal results. The major amount of the water administered was excreted during the day and nocturnal excretion fell to normal levels (Fig. 18).

According to Völker (1927) there is a connection between the course of normal urine excretion and an inner rhythmic process. In comparative experiments carried out in Hamberg and Northern Iceland, he succeeded in proving the hypothesis, still disputed at the time, of an inner rhythm based on local time. The test subjects were examined under invariable experimental conditions (confinement to bed, standardized intake of water and food, etc.). The customary rhythm of water excretion was retained even if the subjects altered their sleep-waking patterns. Völker demonstrated that this body-based rhythm of vital processes also applied to temperature and basal metabolism as well as to pulse and blood pressure.

By using a modified water stress test (based on Gerritzen 1938), Remler (1948) too found inverse water excretion with nocturia in half of his blind experimental subjects. Corroborating the studies of Hollwich (1948), von Schumann (1953), using the Volhard water shock, discovered a lowered four-hour value and an increased nocturnal value (nocturia). As opposed to those who became blind at an early age but who re-

Fig. 16. Top: An 87-year-old patient who gradually reached a state of virtual blindness over a period of ten years as a result of cataracts on both eyes. Note the bloated appearance. Bottom: The same patient three weeks later after cataract surgery. Note the general revitalization and facial tautening resulting from a clinically observed general elimination of fluids.

tained low vision (i.e., ranging from those able to recognize hand movements to those able to count the number of fingers held up) and as opposed to those who became blind later in life (usually with a greater degree of vestigial vision), those who became totally blind when young (amaurosis) displayed the greatest deviations. Fuchs (1953) reports the same results from his studies of ten persons who became totally blind when young, ten who became practically blind when young, and 14 who became practically blind when older. Wassner (1954) studied diuresis in 21 blind children after the Volhard water shock finding a markedly delayed water excretion in the case of 13 who had become blind early, whereas the group retaining more vision showed slighter deviations.

Lobban and Tredre (1964) likewise noted nocturia in 27 totally blind persons and, in addition, a disturbance in their rhythm of excreting sodium and chloride. Jendralsky (1951) reports on his single observation of a case of diabetes insipidus in a person blind

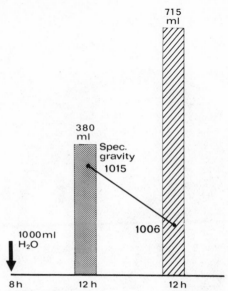

Fig. 18. The Volhard water balance test before and after cataract surgery. In this test water excretion for a four-hour period was measured in patients who had been blind for years as a result of cataracts in both eyes. Before cataract surgery (in the blind state) the four-hour value was lower, after surgery (complete photoperception) normal water excretion was found. Shaded bar, before surgery; hatched bar, after surgery.

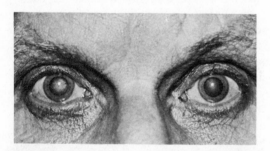

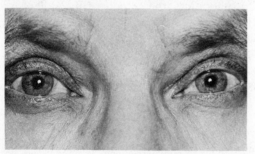

Fig. 17. Top: A patient with cataracts in both eyes. Only a minimal amount of light can penetrate the eyes through the extremely opaque lenses. Bottom: The same patient seen after surgery to remove both opaque lenses. Unhindered entry of light into the eye.

as a result of cataracts on both eyes. After the cataracts were removed and the normal entry of light into the eyes was restored, water excretion became normal.

The change in the rhythm of diuresis has been traced to a reduced efficacy of adiuretin secreted principally during the night by the posterior pituitary lobe. The varying pattern of urine excretion in those with sight and those who are blind becomes clear above all when the water stress test is combined with the injection of the hormone of the posterior pituitary lobe containing antidiuretic hormone (ADH)* (Hollwich 1948). In the case of control subjects with vision, the four-hour figure is reduced by half while the specific gravity remains high; in the case of the blind, there is only a slight reduction of

*ADH determines the concentration power of the kidneys.

ten percent in urine excretion but a sharp drop in specific gravity.

Hofmann-Credner (1953) influenced diuresis by the use of flicker lighting after the Volhard water shock. They found a marked inhibition of urine excretion despite a rise in the kidney's glomerular filtrate. The rise in the *ADH* plasma level is interpreted as the diencephalon's stimulus response to the flicker lighting, as a result of which the antidiuretic hormone (ADH) is excreted.

Electrolyte Balance

Closely connected with water excretion through the kidney is the regulation of electrolyte metabolism. The first report on the diurnal rhythm of electrolyte excretion in healthy people was published after World War I.

Norn's findings (1929)—based mainly on experiments carried out on himself—revealed that when he measured the kidney's excretion of potassium, sodium, and chloride hourly, there were lower amounts during the day than at night. Electrolyte excretion revealed the smallest amounts in the early morning hours, rising then in the course of the morning to reach its highest point in the early afternoon. Norn found this to be most pronounced in potassiun excretion. If the experimental subject slept during the day, then the excretionary pattern was reversed. He said, "The rhythm exhibited is (consequently) determined by the natural change between the day's activity and the night's inactivity or sleep." Campbell and Webster (1922a,b) also believe that the alteration in excretionary rhythm is connected with the alteration in the sleep-waking rhythm.

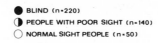

● BLIND (n=220)
◗ PEOPLE WITH POOR SIGHT (n=140)
○ NORMAL SIGHT PEOPLE (n=50)

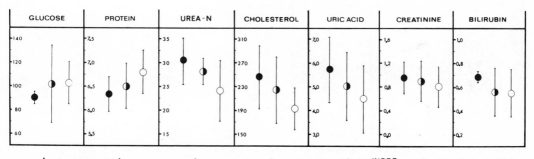

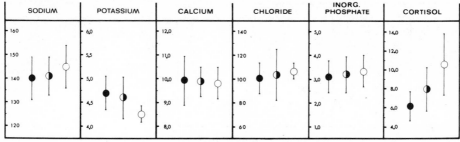

Fig. 19. Mean values, standard deviation, and significance of changes of metabolites (serum) in 220 "practically blind" subjects and 14 subjects with severely impaired vision compared with 50 subjects with normal vision. The blind subjects had significantly lower serum levels of glucose, protein, sodium, chloride, inorganic phosphate and cortisol, and significantly higher levels of nonprotein N, cholesterol, uric acid, creatinine, bilirubin, and calcium.

Manchester (1933) proved that the diurnal rhythm of sodium and potassium is also maintained with fasting and going without fluids on the one hand and with a water intake of approximately two liters on the other. Menzel (1950, 1952) described the rhythmic excretion of chlorine and several organic substances, at the same time pointing out the possible significance of varying rhythms for the differential diagnosis of illnesses. Doe et al (1956) likewise found an excretionary rhythm for sodium and potassium, with the excretion of potassium closely correlated with corticoid excretion.

Bartter and Delea (1962) also saw a diurnal rhythm in the urinary excretion of sodium and potassium in a group of female experimental subjects. Bresnik and Hohenegger (1967) observed a continuous decrease in calcium excretion from a matutinal maximum to a nocturnal minimum. The maximum amount of phosphate excretion took place at night.

Mills (1964) reports on a 105-day-long confinement in a cave in constant darkness. The speleologist used a watch and spoke once a day with someone outside; thus, he was not completely isolated from external influences (social indicators of time). The only thing that was completely eliminated was the physiological day-night sequence in the form of an alternation between light and darkness. A sleep-waking rhythm of somewhat more than 24 hours ensued; potassium excretion in the urine followed this rhythm. The rhythm of urinary excretion of sodium and chloride remained constant for a period of over two months, but then became completely irregular. Within three days after the termination of this experiment in constant darkness, all rhythms became normal again.

Lobban (1965) reports on the amounts of

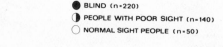

● BLIND (n=220)
◖ PEOPLE WITH POOR SIGHT (n=140)
○ NORMAL SIGHT PEOPLE (n=50)

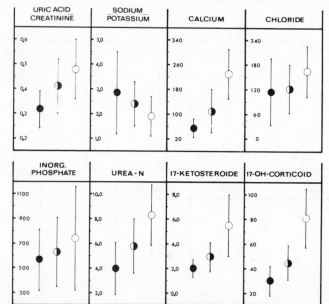

Fig. 20. Changes in metabolites (urinary output). In blind subjects the urine shows an increase in the sodium/potassium ratio as well as lowered values for calcium, chloride, inorganic phosphate, urea-nitrogen, 17-ketosteroids 17-hydroxycorticoids and a fall in the uric acid/creatinine ratio.

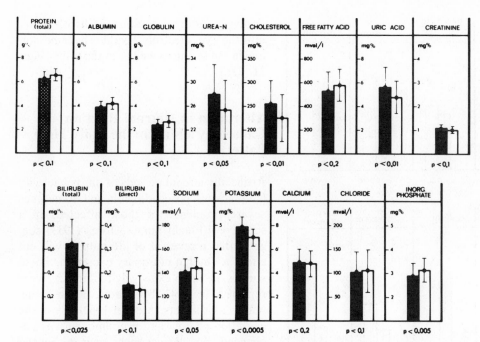

Fig. 21. Percentage changes in metabolic values in the serum of 110 cataract patients before (blind) and after (normal sighted) cataract surgery. Postoperatively, there was a rise in the serum levels of sodium, chloride, phosphate, protein, glucose, and cortisol as well as a fall in the serum levels of potassium, calcium, urea-N, cholesterol, free fatty acids, uric acid, creatinine, and bilirubin. The changes were statistically significant (p .02) in the case of potassium, cholesterol, free fatty acids, uric acid, bilirubin, glucose and cortisol. Shaded bar, before surgery; open bar, after surgery.

electrolyte excretion in the blind. For a period of 24 hours she kept a record of the water and electrolyte excretion of ten blind males. In this study, only the group of five totally blind persons demonstrated—simultaneously with the nocturia already discovered by Hollwich (1948) by using Volhard's stress tests—a shift in the excretion of chloride and sodium to the afternoon. Potassium amplitudes were reduced whereas the rhythm in general was unaffected. In further studies by Lobban and Tredre (1967), 27 totally blind persons exhibited considerable temporal deviations in the amounts of water, sodium, and chloride excreted. Thirty-four persons who became blind between the ages of 12 and 61 but were still able to distinguish between light and dark demonstrated the same quantity of excretion as normal-sighted individuals. Nine older blind persons deviated temporally in their diuresis rhythm

from the rest of the group but not from comparable test subjects with sight.

Simenhoff's study (1968) agrees with Lobban and Tredre's findings that when light-dark perception is present, a normal excretory rhythm is maintained. Upon the incidence of total blindness, the rhythms were altered or completely missing; in the case of congenital amaurosis a complete reversal of the cycle occurred.

Tromp and Bouma (1967) as well as Hollwich and Dieckhues (1967a, 1971b,c) published comparative studies on the total amounts of electrolyte excretion in the urine over a 24-hour period. In their study of 41 boys aged 6 to 18 (14 with amaurosis, 8 with perception of light, and 19 with severe visual impairment), Tromp and Bouma (1967) report an increased amount of sodium excreted in the urine.

Hollwich and Dieckhues (1967a, 1971b,

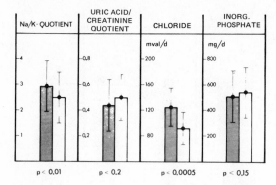

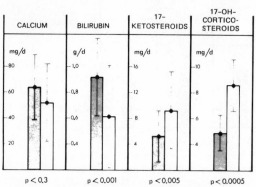

Fig. 22.   Percentage changes in metabolic values in urine in 110 cataract patients before (blind) and after (normal sighted) cataract surgery. Postoperatively, there was a rise in the 17-ketosteroid and 17-OH-corticosteroid excretion in the urine as well as a fall in the excretion of calcium, chloride and bilirubin. The differences were significant (p .02) in the case of the Na/K ratio, and for chloride, bilirubin, 17-ketosteroids, and 17-OH-corticosteroids. Shaded bar, before surgery; open bar, after surgery.

c), in studying 360 visually impaired patients (220 of them virtually blind) in comparison with 50 persons with normal vision, found alterations in the electrolyte balance in the form of an adrenal cortical insufficiency: lowered amounts of sodium, chloride, and inorganic phosphate, and a slightly increased potassium level appeared in the serum. In the urine from a 24-hour period, sodium excretion and the sodium-potassium quotient were increased, in keeping with Tromp's findings. The amounts of calcium, chloride, and inorganic phosphate were reduced (Figs. 19, 20). The same alterations were found in 110 cataract patients who were virtually blind before surgery. Postop-

eratively, after restoration of light's entry into the eye, electrolyte values became normal in the serum as well as in the urine (Figs. 21, 22).

Alteration in Diurnal Rhythm Caused by a Shift in the Daily Time Pattern

Artificially altered periods of diurnal activity have always posed difficult and sometimes severe problems for those affected. In a study of 10 night nurses, Jores (1933) suggests that a reversal of life pattern will not alter the rhythm of urinary excretion. These studies, devoted exlusively to diuresis, were repeated in 1941 ·by Hauff, again using nurses as subjects (Menzel 1962). Even the excretion of urea and urobilinogen was unchanged, i.e., less at night than during the day, in spite of night work and a meal eaten at midnight. Norn (1929) discovered that a night watchman, after six weeks of night duty, did experience a reversal in his diurnal rhythm of sodium, potassium, and chloride excretion.

Experiments that artificially alter the length of the day and the resulting influence on human circadian rhythm have elicited strong interest on the part of all investigators. Mills and Stanbury (1952) already established the persistence of the 24-hour rhythm of water and electrolyte excretion in the case of five subjects who experienced a sleep-waking rhythm of 12 hours for the two days they spent in a basement. We know today from the work of Aschoff et al (1969, 1970, 1973, 1974) that a deviation from the autonomic 24-hour rhythm occurs only when all time indicators are completely eliminated.

Lewis and Lobban (1954) observed the diuresis rhythm of an expedition in Spitsbergen. The eight members of this expedition experienced a 22-hour day in shared isolation for six weeks during the polar summer. The individual members exhibited various reactions to the 22-hour rhythm of work. Almost all of them exhibited a continuation of the endogenic 24-hour rhythm of water excretion, although the 22-hour environmental rhythm and other disturbing factors which it was not possible to identify more specifically seemed to superimpose themselves. Seven of the experimental subjects displayed marked nocturia, especially when their period of sleep coincided with their local time at home.

In a further study, Lewis et al (1956) report on electrolyte excretion during the 22-hour days. For seven of the experimental subjects the existence of the 24-hour potassium rhythm was clearly preserved. For some subjects there were indications of temporary complete disassociation of the diurnal rhythm from that of electrolyte excretion.

In an experiment by Mills and Thomas (1957), a subject who had been on duty as a night watchman for four weeks maintained an unchanged potassium rhythm. The diurnal rhythm of sodium and chloride was also maintained although only slightly altered. Phosphate excretion, on the other hand, did not reveal the usual sharp drop in the early morning but in late evening instead.

Lobban (1963) investigated workers on the night shift in a mine on Spitsbergen. The workers lived mostly in groups in camps; the community's activity conformed to the shift pattern. According to this plan, the shift schedule of each worker remained unchanged for the entire year. In this way, factors of the social environment were reduced to a minimum and thus could not disturb adaptation to the unusual working hours. At monthly intervals, Lobban measured water and potassium excretion in order to study the influence of the change of natural light patterns: the periods of constant darkness in winter, the periods of light and darkness in spring and fall, and those of constant daylight in the summer. For six night shift workers the rhythm of potassium excretion maintained itself well for six months, demonstrating a correlation with the activity pattern of the experimental subject. The highest excretory rate occurred between midnight and 8 A.M. for those be-

ginning work at 4 P.M. The diuresis rhythm during the winter months of constant darkness proved to be markedly abnormal. The regular diurnal rhythm did not reappear until the spring months; it was dissociated, however, from the potassium rhythm. In May, with its constant daylight, maximal rates occurred between 8 A.M. and 4 P.M. The author concluded from this that the six miners on the night shift reacted like "nocturnal animals" with regard to their excretion of potassium and like "diurnal animals" with regard to their diurnal rhythm.

Sharp (1960a) reports on an expedition in Spitsbergen: the six participants experienced an astonishingly exact reversal of diuresis, pH value, potassium and sodium excretion, and of the specific gravity of their urine as a result of the day-night reversal occasioned by their work (made possible by the conditions of the polar summer). This inversion was complete six days after the beginning of the reversed work schedule. A further stipulation of the experiment (1960b) required the participants in the expedition to remain in their darkened tents for three hours after being awakened. This procedure caused a reduction in the diurnal peak of diuresis and in sodium and potassium excretion with a corresponding increase in nocturnal values. On the basis of his research, Sharp posits the conclusion that the diurnal rhythm of diuresis and sodium and potassium excretion is controlled by a single dominant factor whose nature, however, is not known.

Lobban gives a detailed report on electrolyte and water balance disturbances under conditions of polar summer in Spitsbergen and among Eskimos. In experiments lasting six weeks, when there was a scarcely discernible difference in brightness between day and night, Lobban (1960) found the following: the experimental subjects were provided with wristwatches according to the group they belonged to; the watches of some indicated a "day" of 22 hours, the watches of the others one of 27 hours. All activities were conducted as usual within this abnormal time frame, and urine was also collected. In most cases the diuresis rhythm adapted itself to the new division of time without great difficulty; the rhythm of potassium excretion, however, appeared very slowly, if at all. During the 22-hour day, only one out of eight subjects became adapted; during the 27-hour day, two persons exhibited good adaptation. In contrast to water excretion, which adapted well to a changed rhythm, the rhythm of potassium excretion retained its original frequency.

Further series of experiments in this area were carried out by Simpson and Lobban (1967), this time with a 21-hour day. It was not until after five weeks that the shortened day-night alternation brought about an adaptation in the rhythm of corticosteroid and potassium excretion. An astonishing subphenomenon also took place: if an artificial "day" occurred at the time of periods of deep sleep at the subject's own home, then a very slow adaptation resulted. This observation indicates that the 24-hour rhythm is fundamental to the excretory rhythms. Furthermore, these studies confirm Lobban's (1960) postulated hypothesis of two different control mechanisms for the regulation of these rhythms: the hypothalamic-hypophysial axis for water and salt and the adrenal cortex for potassium.

After these surveys of participants in expeditions and those with nighttime work it was a logical step to study the inhabitants of the Arctic regions themselves for their endogenic rhythms. Stated briefly, Lobban (1967) found such a high number of abnormalities in the excretionary rhythm of inhabitants of the Arctic that an average excretionary pattern for the native population was much harder to establish than for a control group of eight inhabitants of temperate zones. In a comparison of the relative amplitude of the rhythm of potassium excretion, the European control group displayed the largest amplitudes, followed by the Indians during the polar summer, then by the Indians during the polar winter, and finally by the Eskimos.

According to Lobban, ethnological differences and differences in age, activity, and customs do not adequately explain these findings. She contends that the normal daily alternation of light and darkness in the environment is necessary not only for the maintenance of kidney rhythm but is also a causal factor for its establishment in early childhood. In 1972 this author reported on studies she undertook 16 years after her first experiments with Arctic Indians. In the first of these (Lobban 1967), the Indians in winter camp exhibited an excretory rhythm with lesser amplitude and temporal increase in comparison with European control subjects. Moreover, there were no differences noted based on sex or age. In a second study of a group of Indians closely related to the first one, she found that they had completely changed their life style and had assumed "modern" ways of life. This time her findings were almost completely the same as in the cases of the control subjects; however, the adults—especially the older Indians—continued to show a distinct time lag.

Krieger et al (1969) studied circadian periodicity of steroids and electrolytes under differing light conditions. Urine samples were collected at four-hour intervals from two healthy subjects who were hospitalized for several weeks in order to determine the effect on electrolyte excretion of a normal light-day rhythm, of a normal day with constant light, and of an inverted sleep rhythm with constant light. The authors discovered a weak correlation between electrolyte excretion and periods of sleep. In the experiment with the inverted sleep pattern, the rhythm of potassium excretion showed a distinctively irregular pattern in contrast to that of the normal day with constant light. Thus, sleeping conditions appear to have a stronger effect on circadian rhythm than periods of darkness.

Alteration in Diurnal Rhythm Caused by Rapid Change of Location

Abruptly occurring time shifts have reached problem proportions for those affected, especially since the introduction of mass air travel. Physical and mental efficiency, especially that of the flight crew, are threatened by severe stress.

Gerritzen (1962) attempted to determine the maximum time required for electrolyte excretion and diuresis to adapt to local time after a rapid time change of five hours between Amsterdam and New York. At the same time, he was also interested in finding out to what extent the disharmony between endogenic rhythm and local time is responsible for the symptoms of disturbance caused by rapid time change. Immediately after the time shift an abnormality in the diurnal excretory rhythm of all electrolytes occurred: amplitude decreased and even after 4 days normal amplitude had not been reestablished, but shifted to the "correct" point in local time. Although it could be assumed that the experimental subjects had not yet completely adapted themselves to local time in New York, it was still remarkable that all rhythms were restored to normal immediately after the return flight. When a flight was immediately followed by a return flight, there was a severe disturbance in excretory rhythm. This was not sufficient, however, to bring about an immediate return to normal rhythm in local Amsterdam time. Gerritzen concluded from this that a flight accompanied by time change causes greater disturbances and alterations in diurnal rhythm than a return to place of origin, especially when the organism is not yet completely adapted to the foreign day–night pattern.

LaFontaine et al (1967) conducted their studies on flight crews on the Paris to Anchorage route. They came to the conclusion that a relatively short stay in Alaska of 20 hours with a time change of 11 hours is not enough to have any lasting effect on the circadian rhythms under study. There was only a slight reduction in the amplitudes of diuresis, of sodium, potassium, and corticoid excretion and negligible disturbances during flight. Upon returning, however, immediate restoration of preflight rhythms occurred. From these studies it can be deduced that if the return flight takes place by the next day, the organism continues to operate according to its local time even on long

flights involving time changes. The authors do not consider what effect longer stays involving time change have on biologic rhythms.

Conroy and Mills (1970) studied a family of three on a flight from Winnipeg to Manchester. After the flight, the excretory rhythm of potassium occurred irregularly, without the recognizable pattern of a sinus rhythm; complete adaptation to local time was attained only after a week had passed. Readaptation after the return flight occurred within a similar period of time. Sodium excretion followed an even more irregular pattern than potassium excretion. In these experiments an immediate reversal in phosphate excretion was observed, i.e., the matutinal decrease adapted itself to local time but did not attain a sinusoid curve with amplitudes in a 12-hour rhythm.

Continuing his studies on the effect of time changes on intercontinental flights, Gerritzen (1966) subjected four groups of five students each to strictly standardized experimental conditions: hourly intake of fluid and food, hourly collection of urine for two to three days. He discovered that under these conditions the rhythmic excretion of water and electrolytes can be suppressed by means of light reversal. On the other hand, the creation by means of light manipulation of maximum excretion at a different definitive time of day than that determined by endogenic rhythm is not possible for short time periods. The goal of his research proved to be unattainable: shifting circadian periodicity by means of light manipulation in order to facilitate more rapid adaptation of the flight crew to the foreign local time and thus to maintain their physical and mental efficiency.

Diurnal Rhythm in Children

Hellbrügge (1960, 1965) traced, among other things, the development, formation, and stabilization of a 24-hour rhythm in infants from birth. Independently of fluid intake, urine excretion reveals a 24-hour periodicity as early as the fourth week, whereas potassium and sodium excretion was not evident until the age of three and one-half months. In addition, his studies of phosphate and creatinine excretion did not demonstrate a day–night periodicity until the fourth month. In the case of creatinine and chloride excretion it was not until the 16th month that a reasonably significant difference between day and night amounts was found. According to Hellbrügge, the infant possesses an innate circadian rhythm, at the basis of which is an endogenic, self-induced fluctuation. Depending upon the organ's state of maturity, this endogenic frequency is supposed to be transformed into a 24-hour periodicity. In his view, effective time indicators are, above all, the effects of temperature and periodically recurring stimuli connected with the baby's care as well as social time indicators. It remains unclear why he excludes a time-indicating function of the light–darkness alternation in spite of the very early functioning of the energetic portion of the visual pathway, and this mainly on the basis of measurements of electric skin resistance and the periodicity of epidermal mitoses.

In her most recent studies of Eskimo children (1974) during all four seasons, Lobban found a much more distinct formation of renal excretionary rhythm than in the case of their parents, especially in spring and fall when light serves as a natural time indicator. In the polar summer, the fact that their activity takes place throughout the whole day is probably the cause of the complete disorganization of rhythms. Specifically, potassium rhythm developed two secretory peaks, a situation also found in earliest infancy (Hellbrügge 1960). In the constant darkness of polar winter, the orderly social environment and diurnal periodicity in school appear to be responsible for the maintenance of renal excretory rhythms, which is not the case for the parents of the Eskimo children.

Forecast

The most recent studies of circadian rhythm in the renin-angiotensine-aldosterone system utilizing chromatographic and radioimmunological methods are of great promise for further clarification of the endogenic regulatory mechanisms, in particular of the renal excretory rhythm (Breuer et al 1974; Grim et al 1974; Kaulhausen et al 1974; Vagnucci et al 1974; Katz et al 1975; Kowarski et al 1975). To be sure, these studies are conducted primarily for clinical purposes, but they can also be significant for further clarification of the cause of circadian rhythms.

7
Light and Blood Count

Blood, according to Goethe in *Faust I*, is a "special kind of juice." Blood is of manifold significance to the organism: its functions are partly autonomous, partly of an intermediary nature; the bloodstream serves as the transmitting agent to and from the cells and organs. Furthermore, the blood carries out the exchange of hormones and other substances regulating the organs and cell function.

But blood also has an autonomous nature. Its corpuscular elements are living cells, each category of which has its own structure, metabolism, and functions. The composition of blood is subject to constant change, even under normal circumstances. It also follows from the fact that blood is involved so closely with the whole organism that a change in blood count accompanies almost all ailments and abnormalities of the organism.

Red Blood Cell Count

Numerous mechanisms are responsible for the direction and regulation of erythropoie-sis. Thus, the autonomic nervous system plays a role in the transmission of red cells to the body's periphery, especially in cases of emergency. Lack of oxygen is a specific stimulus for the formation of red blood cells. A special agent stimulating erythropoiesis is erythropoietin, which is formed (or at least is activated) in the kidneys. When there is reduced need, normally the number of erythrocytes decreases due to a slowdown in production or, less frequently, due to hemolysis. There is still uncertainty concerning the processes that contribute to the constant maintenance of normal cell counts in the peripheral blood.

The role of light in the formation of blood is not clearly evaluated in the relevant literature and is frequently even strictly denied. Most studies merely serve the purpose of a broad orientation and are so heterogeneous that a generally valid statement is scarcely possible. To some extent, older experimental methods, which do not always utilize the results of recent innovations, are involved here.

Earlier researchers (Graffenberger 1893; Marti 1897; Schoenenberger 1898; Grober and Sempell 1919; Clark 1921; Hobert 1923; Miles and Laurens 1926a,b) were not able to give persuasive evidence of light's effect on the blood count. The reason for their varying findings might have been errors in method as well as varying experimental conditions, especially those having to do with the duration and amount of exposure to light.

The basic question of whether placing light-adapted animals in complete darkness for an extended period has an effect on the number of their erythrocytes has been investigated repeatedly. Oltramare (1919) found no reduction in erythrocytes in various animals (rabbits, guinea pigs, roosters, doves, frogs, newts, and fish) who spent three months in darkness.

Grober and Sempell (1919) investigated the hemoglobin and erythrocyte values in horses who had spent years in the dark tunnels of coal mines without natural daylight. Illumination consisted solely of isolated, weakly burning carbon filament lamps. They found a uniform reduction in hemoglobin along with a marked increase in erythrocytes. Their assumption was that the excellent care given the animals, the abundant feed, and strenuous work compensated for the absence of daylight so that such a lack, lasting for years, did not cause clear-cut anemia in the mine horses.

In his studies on the influence of "bad air" on general growth, blood counts, and condition of the organs, Cropp (1922) subjected young white rats to darkness, finding no uniform difference between these animals and control animals kept in light. He concluded from this that the absence of light does not have a negative effect on the general development and erythropoiesis of the growing organism.

We owe to Hobert (1923) the first orientative attempt to explain the effect of light in the case of posthemorrhagic anemia. He made two groups of four white mice each anemic by draining off 50 percent of their blood supply. Whereas the mice kept in darkness died after two days, their blood showing a decrease in Hb and erythrocytes, the blood of those kept in daylight regained its original count in two weeks. Ultraviolet irradiation shortened the period of regeneration to nine or ten days.

Häberlein et al (1923) traced the development of hemoglobin content in the blood of ailing urban children who were exposed to the influence of the North Sea climate. The rise in the curve of their progress chart correlates clearly with the length of daily exposure to sunshine. Like Isachsen (1925), Häberlein found the highest hemoglobin levels in the sunny spring and summer months, the lowest levels in the months of November and December with their dearth of sunshine. He explained this by pointing out that the body receives more chemically active radiation by the sea due to the increased reflection of sunshine, just as it does in the high mountains due to the thinner layer of air.

Laquer (1924) deserves mention for his isolated observation: he exposed himself to a mountain climate for one month and, experimenting on himself with the aid of Griesbach's Congo red method, he measured total blood volume, which showed a marked increase in erythrocytes and in the total amount of blood. He does not attribute the decisive effect of the mountain climate to the lower partial pressure of oxygen which had been generally assumed. Since a genuine increase in blood occurs even at the relatively low altitudes of the city of Davos, Switzerland, Laquer sees the very intensive solar radiation as the possible causal agent.

Upon keeping five dogs in constant darkness for nine months, Miles and Laurens (1926a) discovered an initial fall in hemoglobin and erythrocyte levels with subsequent fluctuations levelling off at subnormal levels.

Several authors have dealt with variations in the diurnal rhythm of hemoglobin and erythrocytes in connection with the day–night alternation. In his survey of the literature, Jores (1935a) reports on proven physiological diurnal fluctuations between higher morning levels and lower evening levels of up to half a million erythrocytes.

Renbourn (1947) discovered a continuous fall of hematocrit in rabbits during the course of the day. In humans, hemoglobin content together with hematocrit falls markedly from 7 A.M. until after midnight. In the course of a year, the author found evidence for an increase in blood parameters during the summer.

Unshelm (1968) and Unshelm and Hagemeister (1971) investigated fluctuations related to the time of day in the number of erythrocytes and in hemoglobin content of cows. In accordance with the studies already mentioned, they discovered a maximum in the morning and a minimum in the evening. In the case of hemoglobin content, the day-to-day influence was greater than the factor of the time of day, which agrees with the results obtained by Brown and Goodall (1946), who made the same findings for humans.

A clear contrast to the apparently slight reactive behavior of the blood count of nocturnal rats and mice (Hollwich and Tilgner 1964a) is offered by diurnal birds (Hollwich 1953): seven-week-old roosters were kept in a darkened room for ten weeks during the summer months. The result was pronounced anemia: pale combs and leg skin, general loss of tone, reduction of hemoglobin by half. The eyelids of 20 roosters were subsequently sutured, the eyelids of ten were left open. Both groups—the experimental and control birds—were exposed to sunlight for five days for two hours in the morning and

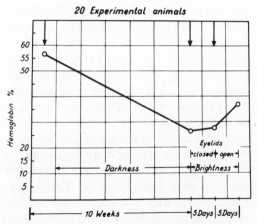

20 Experimental animals

Fig. 24. Behavior of the level of hemoglobin in young chickens after staying in a darkened room, then with sutured eyelids, and finally with reopened eyelids in brightness.

two hours in the afternoon, and hemoglobin levels were then examined. The following picture emerged: light hastened the regeneration of red blood cells when the lids were open but not when they were sewn shut (Figs. 23, 24). The varying behavior of hemoglobin levels in the two groups demonstrates that the full regenerative effect of light becomes active only when it enters the eye. These experiments confirm Heilmeyer's (1942) view: "the old common sense belief that sunlight promotes the production of blood appears clearly in regeneration experiments, i.e., when a higher efficiency than usual is demanded of the bone marrow."

Blood Sedimentation Reaction

Blood sedimentation is dependent on the protein spectrum and fibrinogen content of blood and, thus, to the extent that pathological factors can be excluded, is an indirect indicator of the way the former vary according to the time of day. There is a tendency for total protein content in humans to rise between 8 A.M. and noon, to fall in the afternoon, and to reach a minimum during the night (Kröger et al 1928; Renbourn 1947;

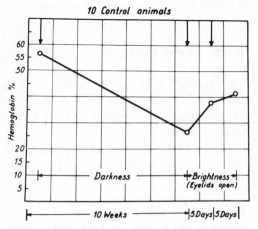

10 Control animals

Fig. 23. Behavior of the level of hemoglobin in control animals after staying first in a darkened room then brought into brightness.

Seaman et al 1965). As early as 1924 Westergren reported pathological daily fluctuations in the blood sedimentation rate (BSR)* of over 20 mm. Katz and Leffkowitz (1928) presumed here a certain parallel to the daily temperature curve. But these authors also did not attribute any special significance to these fluctuations.

To clarify the question of the degree to which there are regular daily fluctuations of blood corpuscles, Jores (1934b, 1935a) conducted experiments, based on Westergren's principle, in which measurements of the sedimentation rate were taken every two hours for 24 hours in normal as well as pathological cases. The results were unequivocal. Extremely regular fluctuations occurred, with an evening peak reaching as much as 50 percent of the normal rate.

Unshelm (1968) found significant daily fluctuations for the hematocrit level in cows with a maximum in the morning and a minimum in the evening. This progressive reduction was interrupted by rises at noon and 4 P.M. Reinberg (1974) reached similar conclusions.

Tromp (1973, 1974) compiled data from blood banks, starting with the assumption that differing geographical spreads and climatic conditions must be reflected in the hematological data of blood donors. He obtained an enormous amount of data in this manner. In a study lasting 18 years, he found that blood sedimentation values in the Netherlands were lowest in winter and highest in summer and were clearly distinguishable from month to month. The blood pigment content was higher in fall and winter than in spring and summer. Short-term fluctuations in sedimentation values are frequently influenced by the blood's fibrinogen level, which rises on very warm days along with the BSR. In Tromp's view, BSR values in healthy male blood donors are dependent mainly on fluctuations in fibrinogen level, which in turn are influenced to a great extent by atmospheric conditions. In addition, with a decrease in the degree of latitude and altitude, the proportion of low BSR values declines. Along with the influence of climate and altitude Tromp discusses an influence of light which can explain the following differing types of blood count: from the equator to the north pole an increasing proportion in low blood sedimentation values and a rise in the content of blood pigment.

A Russian research group was studied during the winter months in the Antarctic (Vencenoscev 1972). A fall in hemoglobin concentration as well as in the number of erythrocytes was seen, but it was under the physiological threshold. By the beginning of the polar summer all the measured elements had become normal again. Vitamin and salt deficiency, cold, alterations of the magnetic field as well as cosmic radiation and annual photo periods are discussed as causes for the change.

In contrast to the red blood corpuscles the leukocytes are nucleate elements, in other words, genuine cells. Granulocytes and monocytes possess the two important qualities of phagocytosis and chemotaxis, which explains their importance in fighting off infective agents. Lymphocytes and plasma cells are responsible for the synthesis of antibodies. This highly important function is performed by specific cells in the lymph nodes, spleen, and reticuloendothelial system of the liver and bone marrow.

White Blood Cell Count

The exposure of organisms to ultraviolet radiation was in its turn a point of departure for investigating the effect of light on the white blood count.

Clark (1921) exposed rabbits to daily ultraviolet radiation; after a rapid drop on the first day he found a sharp increase in leukocytes, specifically in the lymphocyte count. There was a subsequent return to normal values in the course of three weeks. Upon closer investigation, however, she was able

---

* The erythrocyte sedimentation rate is dependent upon a complex of change in the protein balance.

to demonstrate an in part opposite effect in other areas of the spectrum. Hobert (1923) irradiated anemic mice and found an immediate rise in the leukocyte count paralleling the changes in the red blood count already mentioned.

Koenigsfeld (1921) studied the influence of irradiation with artificial sunlight on human metabolism and blood count. He observed a marked effect on the leukocyte and white blood cell counts. This took the form of a considerable increase in the number of leukocytes shortly after irradiation, if it had been prolonged. He places leukocytosis brought about by irradiation on the same level as "digestive leukocytosis" (which we shall return to later). In his view, as in the digestive processes leukocytes are not primarily formed anew, but rather strengthened demands are made secondarily on the leukocytic apparatus and cells are mobilized. Spode (1954a,b, 1955a,b) studied the reaction of the white blood cell count to ultraviolet irradiation of a cutaneous area in the case of an albino rabbit. Depending on the original total leukocyte count, there was either no reaction or a strong one. In the case of low original values there was a rise, in the case of medium values no effect, and with high amounts a drop in the numbers of cells. In the differential blood count, neutrophils always increased whereas lymphocytes always decreased. Daily fluctuations were clearly superimposed upon the course of the curve (we shall return to this later). Similar results were also obtained in experiments involving irradiation with *visible light*. In the behavior of the white blood cells Spode saw a typical stress reaction, such as has often been observed with unspecific stimuli of various kinds. He attributes special significance to the fact that reactions occur such as are generally ascribed only to ultraviolet light, although the active radiation stimulus belongs solely to the *visible portion* of the optic spectrum.

When mice were exposed to short, very intensive photostimuli (5,000 lux white light), Surowiak and Tilgner (1966) observed—along with the expected eosinopenia—altered relations between neutrophils and lymphocytes, to the advantage of the latter. Two weeks of darkness led to a depression of the white blood corpuscles; the effect of strong light after darkness brought the values of the white blood count back to the normal level. The authors attribute this exclusively to the effect of the ocular perception of light.

A relatively large number of publications primarily in the area of human medicine deal with fluctuations, dependent upon the time of day, of the total leukocytes, and above all of the eosinophilic granulocytes. Distinct fluctuations dependent on the time of day in the total leukocyte count in humans have been described by Sabin et al (1925), who observed a regular fluctuation in the leukocyte count at hourly intervals. Shaw (1927) was not able to find this cycle; instead, he discovered two peaks with a higher afternoon value, almost a tidelike behavior.

Diurnal periodicity of leukocyte values was emphatically rejected by Ponder et al (1932), who carried out Sabin's experiments under conditions of light exercise, finding no indication of fluctuations and explaining all such findings as methodological errors. Nevertheless, they could not help but notice that in their series of experiments too an afternoon rise in leukocytes occurred very frequently.

Thereafter, Jores (1934a,b, 1935a) tried carefully to eliminate methodological errors and found a very constant evening peak in the leukocyte count when it was tested hourly. In addition, he studied the question of the degree to which fluctuations in the periphery are merely changes in distribution, discovering that fluctuations in the leukocyte count occur in the blood of the heart as well as the blood of the vena cava inferior—only that the amounts in the peripheral blood are greater. Jores concludes from his studies that leukocytes display a regular rhythm in the peripheral blood, with an invariable increase in the evening hours and a minimum in the morning hours. This means

that the physiological movements of leukocytes can be classified in the category of
diurnally periodic processes.

Bartter et al (1962) found a pronounced
diurnal rhythm for monocytes, polymorphonuclear neutrophils, and lymphocytes. They
saw this as an exact copy of the corticoid
rhythm, in which the number of circulating
lymphocytes falls as the blood levels rise
and the number of polymorphonuclear leukocytes rises. *These peripheral fluctuations
in blood cells depend on the secretory peaks
of the corticosteroids.* In their investigations
of rhythm in obstetrics and gynecology, Malek et al (1962a,b) observed among other
things the behavior of leukocytes. Total leukocyte count, polymorphonuclear neutrophils, and staff cells displayed a maximum
during the day and a minimum at night,
whereas eosinophils and lymphocytes exhibited, as expected, a reverse pattern. The
authors regarded this curve, which they
found in hospitalized pregnant women
shortly before delivery, as significant for laboratory measurements rather than as the
expression of a diurnal rhythm controlled by
light.

Sharp (1960c) was able to demonstrate a
direct effect of light in the case of the healthy
human. Varying the daily physiological pattern, he exposed his experimental subjects
to an additional three-hour period of darkness after they had awakened and begun
light exercise. This had the effect of sharply
reducing physiological eosinopenia and lymphopenia. After exposure to light there was
a further prolonged drop in both types of
blood cells. The diurnal minimum occurred
belatedly during the three hours spent in
darkness. Under unchanging conditions of
constant light during the polar summer in
Spitsbergen (1960b), lymphocytes and baso-
phil periodicity proved to be related to the
sleep-waking rhythm. By reversing this
rhythm, inverse diurnal rhythms of these
blood cells occurred after a three to six-day
period of adjustment.

Continuing earlier studies on fluctuations
of various hormonal and metabolic parameters, Hollwich and Dieckhues (1973) investi-

gated diurnal fluctuations in blood count as
related to the perception of light on the part
of the blind and of control subjects with
normal sight. Blind people, whose perception of light was totally lacking or sharply
reduced, exhibited a diurnal rhythm which
deviated from the norm. Furthermore, these
authors were the first to point out that the
absolute number of leukocytes in the practically blind is lowered in a most significant
fashion. In the differential blood count the
number of lymphocytes and neutrophils in
the blind was also reduced. Reticulocytes
and hematocrit value behaved the same as
for leukocytes. All diurnal values of the
blood count were lower than in the cases of
those with normal sight. Studies of cataract
patients before (practically blind) and after
(sight restored) surgery (Figs. 25A, B)
yielded the same results. The absence of
photostimulation of the eye leads—as studies by the same researchers (1966, 1967a)

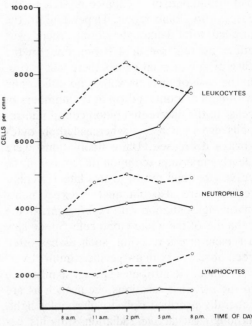

Fig. 25A. Diurnal fluctuations in blood count
(median value and range of fluctuations) in blind
and normal-sighted people. The normal matutinal
rise of leukocytes, neutrophils, and lymphocytes
does not occur in the blind. In addition, the absolute number of blood cells is significantly lower
in the blind (t-test: .0005 p .01).

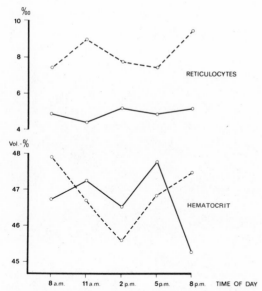

Fig. 25B. For reticulocytes the normal sighted have a dual-peaked course of curve. The blind exhibit an inverse behavior with a lowering of the absolute number of reticulocytes. The blind and normal sighted have a different behavior of hematocrit. The normal course of the curve with a fall until noon and a subsequent rise is only weakly distinguishable in the blind. The hematocrit value is significantly lower for the blind. Solid line, blind (n = 25); broken line, normal sighted (n = 25).

using the Thorn test (1948) indicate—to reduced pituitary activity due to a secondary insufficiency of the adrenal cortex. This in turn causes a decrease in total leukocytes and a shift in the differential blood count.

Thrombocytes

The formation of thrombocytes begins in the giant cells of the bone marrow, the megakaryocytes. The blood platelets are extraordinarily sensitive structures whose exact measurement causes certain difficulties. It is understandable that data on the number of thrombocytes can vary greatly, since we are confronted here with extremely fragile elements. This appears to be the main reason why the behavior of thrombocytes exposed to light has been studied relatively little.

Laurens and Sooy (1924) studied the thrombocyte count in three groups of rats

who 1) had been exposed to the sun, 2) exposed to daylight, or 3) had been kept in darkness. The latter exhibited the lowest values, the animals who had been in the sun the highest ones, whereas the count for the rats who had been exposed to daylight was in the middle.

The first information concerning physiological diurnal fluctuations in thrombocyte counts in humans was provided by Kranzfeld (1925), who measured the blood platelet count every two hours in healthy women in the middle of their menstrual cycle. The author of this study reported a rise until 4 P.M. and a subsequent drop until 10 P.M. Sabin and co-workers (1925) reported finding similar behavior for thrombocytes and leuko-

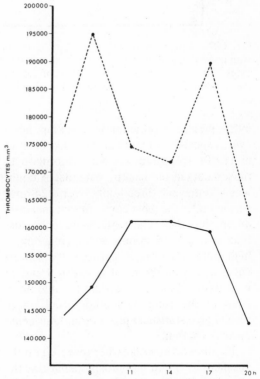

Fig. 26A. Comparison of rhythm in thrombocytes between normal and blind people during the diurnal phase of the 24-hour period. Thrombocytes of people with normal vision show marked diurnal changes. In blind persons this rhythm is disturbed. The amplitude is lowered and the absolute number of thrombocytes in the blood is reduced. Broken line, normal sight (n = 250); solid line, blind.

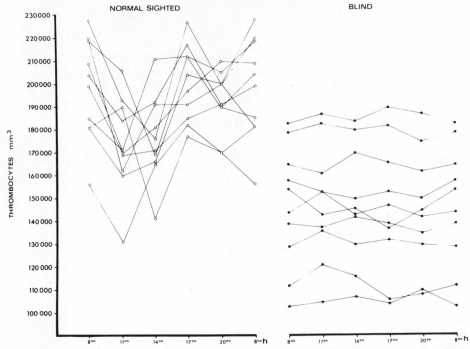

Fig. 26B. Circadian thrombocyte rhythm (individual curves) in the blind and in 10 persons with normal ocular light perception. Individual pattern of the diurnal fluctuation of thrombocytes in the two categories: Diminution of the diurnal rhythm in the blind with a reduction of the total number of thrombocytes in the blood.

cytes; precise information was lacking, however, especially numerical data. Goldeck et al (1950) measured periodic thrombocyte movements in ten healthy patients. A count was taken every three hours over a 24-hour period under the most constant external conditions possible. Their studies reveal a distinct rise around noon, usually reaching a high point at 3 P.M., whereas the lowest value occurs in the night between 9 and 11 P.M. Even taking into account the margin of error of the counting method used, these results give statistical proof of an *endogenic 24-hour* rhythm.

In connection with earlier research on the absence of matutinal eosinopenia in the blind (Hollwich and Tilgner 1964b, 1965; Hollwich and Dieckhues 1966), Hollwich and Dieckhues (1972b) investigated the question of the diurnal thrombocyte rhythm in 250 blind persons. After they received light, the matutinal behavior of thrombo-

cytes was measured in 50 cataract patients before and after removal of the opaque lens. Like the diurnal eosinophilic fluctuations, thrombocytes also normally show a diurnal rhythm reaching a maximum at 8 A.M. with a subsequent drop until midnight, interrupted by a second peak around 5 P.M. Starting at midnight, there is in turn a gradual increase until the maximum in the early morning hours. In contrast to the thrombocyte count in persons with normal sight, the matutinal decline does not take place in the blind. Rather, their thrombocytes display an inverse behavior with a matutinal rise reaching a maximum in the afternoon. The two daily peaks cannot be found in the blind either. Moreover, the absolute thrombocyte count in the blind is also significantly lower than in those with normal sight (Figs. 26A, B). These studies reveal the different behavior of thrombocytes in the blind and in those with normal sight.

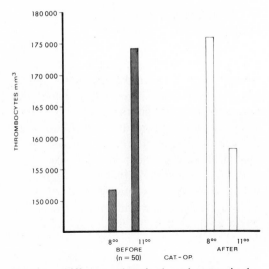

Fig. 27. Different values in thrombocytes in the morning before and after cataract operation for 50 persons. The characteristic morning decrease between 8:00 and 11:00 A.M. in people with normal sight is absent in cataract patients. Postoperatively with regained restoration of ocular light perception the normal decrease is regained.

In cataract patients with diminished ocular perception of light due to opaque lenses, the abnormal matutinal rise in thrombocytes between 8 and 11 A.M. becomes normal after surgery. After free passage of light to the interior of the eye was restored, thrombocytes showed a regular decline between 8 and 11 A.M., just as in those with normal sight (Fig. 27). Further, a rise in the absolute thrombocyte count was exhibited postoperatively after restoration of normal ocular perception of light. With nutritional and environmental conditions remaining constant, postoperative variations in thrombocyte count in the same test person can only be attributed to the restored passage of light to the retina.

Because of the possibility of studying virtually blind cataract patients pre- and postoperatively, Hollwich and Dieckhues (1972b) were in a position to conduct a carefully directed experiment which might be

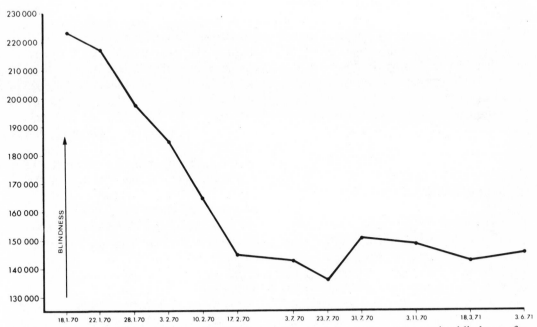

Fig. 28. Decrease of thrombocytes after blindness. The chart shows the postoperative blindness of a 67-year-old female patient in her remaining good eye. In the first four weeks of her blindness the thrombocyte count decreased slowly by approximately 40 percent. During the following time (period of observation 1 year) subnormal values of the thrombocyte level such as are characteristic for the blind developed.

reproduced at any time. Analogous to the movement of eosinophils, ocular photostimuli affect the function of the adrenal cortex and thus the rhythm and extent of thrombocyte fluctuations. The authors were also able to demonstrate the reverse process in the behavior of the thrombocyte count in a patient who had become acutely blind. In the study, a 67-year-old woman had lost the sight of one eye as a child in an accident while playing and lost sight in the other eye due to an intraocular infection; as a consequence she was practically blind. The thrombocyte count was taken beginning on the day she became blind, and thrombocyte values consistently lower than normal were found. After four weeks the values attained the level of thrombocytopenic values characteristic for the blind (Hollwich and Dieckhues 1972b) (Fig. 28). This observation reveals the significance of intact ocular perception of light on thrombocyte fluctuations: if photostimuli are absent, then apparently there is a lack of stimulation to activate the adrenal cortex. The fact that Hollwich and Dieckhues (1972b) were able to stimulate the adrenal cortex in the blind as well as in cataract patients by injections of ACTH and thus cause a drop in thrombocytes points to the correlation of thrombocyte count with adrenal cortical activity. *ACTH therefore had the same effect in this experiment as the ocular perception of light.*

Eosinophilic Blood Cells

Photostimuli also affect the number of eosinophilic cells just as they do other blood cells. Domarus (1931) was probably the first to point out that it was specifically the number of eosinophils which showed considerable diurnal fluctuation. He found that the first matutinal value was always higher than those found in the following hours. Physical activities and food intake had no effect. Domarus attributed the matutinal drop in eosinophils after awakening to the transition between sleep and waking or, in other words,

to the influence of the autonomic nervous system.

Subsequently, Djavid (1935) also found characteristic differences in the absolute eosinophil count measured at different times of day. The relatively high fasting values fall during the morning hours and clearly, and to some extent even considerably, rise again in the course of the afternoon. According to Djavid, there is an independent diurnal fluctuation of eosinophils that is unconnected with illness, age, sex, and life pattern.

In counting eosinophils in the circulating blood at three-hour intervals, Appel (1939) as well as Jores (1934a,b, 1935a, 1938) found a matutinal fall followed by a constant rise in the count lasting till nighttime. To determine the cause of these fluctuations, Appel (1939) first assumed that, as believed earlier, digestion and nutrition played a role here. Experiments with fasting as well as with various diets, however, induced no variation in the diurnal eosinophilic curve. After making studies of night nurses, Appel discovered that it was the sunrise and not the act of awakening which was followed by a fall in eosinophil count, independently of the rhythm of physical activity. Further research showed that the earlier the sun rose, the earlier the fall in the number of eosinophils occurred. From these results of his research, Appel concluded that light has the decisive influence on the 24-hour rhythm of eosinophils.

As proven by experiments on the blind (Hollwich and Tilgner 1964b; Hollwich 1964a,b; Hollwich and Tilgner 1965; Hollwich and Dieckhues 1966, 1968), *the transition between sleep and waking does not have any substantial influence on the matutinal fall of eosinophil cells; rather, it is the ocular perception of light which is responsible for this.*

Photostimuli entering the body via the eye have two marked effects. First, many observations indicate that light entering the eye adapts the endogenically determined adrenal cycle to the physiological light-darkness alternation. Thus, ocular light perception is of indirect significance for the rhythm of the eosinophil count in the peripheral blood. According to Aschoff (1954) and Halberg (1955), it fulfills the function of a time indicator. This view is supported by the fact (among others) that deviations in the rhythm of eosinophils occur after total blindness by double enucleation (Kresbach and Rabel 1954; Landau and Feldmann 1954).

Second, light entering the eye assumes the function of a stress inducer, providing an example of a general adaptive syndrome. The prerequisites for this process are intensive stimulatory levels of light (high intensity of illumination or flicker light) (Figs. 29, 30) and functional efficiency of the eye and neuroendocrine system (Hollwich and Dieckhues 1968).

Ponte and co-workers (1960) obtained similar results when they exposed 15 healthy male adults to intermittent photostimulus and found an eosinophil count 25 percent lower than in the control subjects. The serum electrolytes sodium and potassium, on the other hand, showed no significant change.

In studies of normal levels of eosinophil

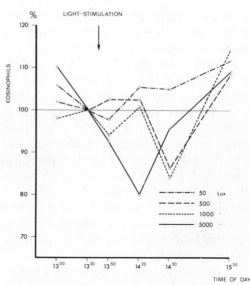

Fig. 30. Changes of eosinophils by light of various intensity in a subject with normal vision. The eosinophil count was measured as light intensity increased. With increase in the lux number, the eosinopenic effect occurs earlier and more distinctly.

count, Fisher and Fisher (1951) discovered a matutinal eosinophil drop, which could also be caused by adrenal extracts.

Doe et al (1956) followed diurnal fluctuations in corticosteroid urine excretion, plasma level, and eosinophil count in 25 healthy males under identical environmental conditions. They found a diurnal eosinophilic curve following the plasma 17-OHCS* level.

Halberg et al (1958) observed the development of diurnal eosinophilic rhythm in six patients who had suffered from hemiplegia as well as from intractable epilepsy since childhood. Hemidecortication was performed on these patients; the diseased cerebral hemisphere and portions of the stem ganglia were removed depending on the extent of the disease. Postoperative observation showed that the diurnal eosinophilic rhythm remained unaffected. The authors conclude from this that the cerebral hemispheres are not necessary for the establishment of this rhythm.

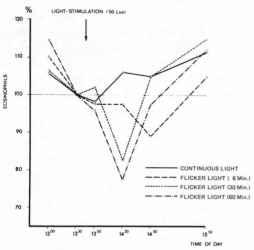

Fig. 29. Changes of eosinophils by flicker light of various frequencies in a subject with normal vision. The eosinophil count was measured when the subject was exposed to various frequencies of flicker light and constant light intensity (50 lux). Increase in the frequency of the flicker light causes a stronger eosinopenic effect which occurs early.

*17-Hydroxycorticosteroid (cortisone, cortisol), an excretory product of cortisol.

In his experiments with healthy test persons, Sharp (1960b,c) found a decrease in matutinal eosinopenia as soon as physical activity was initiated during extension of the period of darkness. In another series of experiments during the polar summer (1960) with constant conditions of exposure to light, food, and work rhythm, a complete reversal in the eosinophilic rhythm occurred just three days after the work rhythm had been shifted by 12 hours. Sharp attributes the fact that these results were often not obtained in earlier research by other authors to the all too frequent presence of disturbing external factors, which assume the functions of time indicators.

Radnot et al (1960, 1964) chose hospitalized patients for their research who, because of extended confinement under similar environmental conditions, could be observed both with and without the effect of light. Under normal light conditions the familiar diurnal eosinophilic curve occurred. Since the nature of their eye treatment already required a binocular bandage, the patients could easily be observed in darkness for long periods. As the length of the period of darkness increased, matutinal eosinopenia decreased until it showed only an insignificant diurnal fluctuation. The authors attribute this effect primarily to the elimination of natural photostimulus.

In diseases of the optic nerve and retina, an impairment of the field of vision can occur to varying degrees. In studying cases of such diseases, Radnot and Wallner (1965) found that exposure to light affected the eosinopenic reaction. Even in cases of severe peripheral impairment of the visual field, they found the matutinal or experimentally inducible drop in eosinophils unchanged when degenerations in pigment were present. If, however, the macula was affected by degeneration; chorioretinitis; or diabetic, hypertonic, or myopic retinopathy; then, depending on the extent of visual deterioration or impairment of the central field of vision, an eosinophilic reaction could no longer be elicited. The authors conclude that the diurnal fluctuation in eosinophil count is dependent on the function of the macula region of the retina and thus can be used to test macula function. This assumption was corroborated by the results of studies of diseases of the optic nerves: normal eosinopenia occurred in all clear-cut, uncomplicated cases of optic neuritis, retrobulbar neuritis, and optic atrophy. This also applied to those cases in which there were severely reduced vision and appreciable central scotoma. The absence of the eosinopenic reaction in macula degeneration when vision is good and central scotoma is slight supports the view that the optic and autonomic functions of the eye are separate, as postulated by Hollwich (1948) in his hypothesis of an "energetic portion of the optic system."

Koleszar (1968) studied the effect of photostimulus on eosinophils in 163 eyes (90 persons) with eye diseases. He also found that in all diseases not accompanied by macula changes, there was no effect on the normal eosinophil reaction, but when the fovea centralis was damaged the photoenergetic reaction did not take place.

Appel and Hansen (1952) conducted studies of the effect of impaired photoperception on the behavior of the diurnal eosinophil curve. They discovered a complete reversal of this curve in totally blind test subjects. In spite of the great dispersion of measured values, they were able to detect a sharp increase in matutinal values (in contrast to the values of those with normal sight) as well as a drop toward evening. Levy and Conge (1953) observed a levelling of the diurnal curve in blind persons (whose blindness had varying causes). The first measurement took place relatively late, at 9 A.M. In contrast to all other researchers mentioned, however, the authors did not find matutinal eosinopenia in test persons with good sight. They found a high initial value almost equal to the evening value.

Landau and Feldmann (1954) studied endogenic matutinal eosinopenia in the blind. They compared the eosinophil count in the early morning hours with the later morning count and ascertained that eosinopenia occurs more markedly in those with normal sight than in the blind.

In a study already mentioned of the effect of unimpaired macula function on eosinophilic reaction, Radnot and Török (1957) also discovered that opacity of the eye media can influence matutinal eosinopenia.

Even though other exogenic stimuli function as synchronizing factors in the movement of eosinophils, there is no doubt that *ocular photostimuli* play the dominant role. This emerges from the studies already cited. In addition, intensive ocular photostimuli can elicit stress reactions. They cause, among other things, an increase in the activity of the adrenal cortex. As hormone secretion increases in the blood, the eosinophil count drops off. Hollwich and Tilgner (1963) found a reduction in eosinophil count in humans and animals after intensive exposure to light (Fig. 31); after the use of flicker light, Ponte et al (1961) found the same in adults and Kriens (1956) found the same in children.

In detailed series of experiments by Hollwich and Tilgner (1963b, 1964) and Hollwich and Dieckhues (1966, 1967b, 1968, 1972a,b,

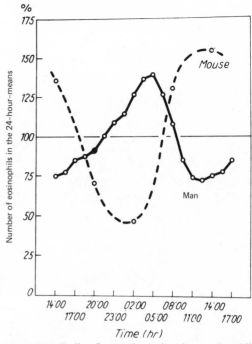

Fig. 32. Daily fluctuations in the eosinophil count in man and in mouse (diagram of the values of v. Domarus, Halberg, and of research conducted by Hollwich and Tilgner).

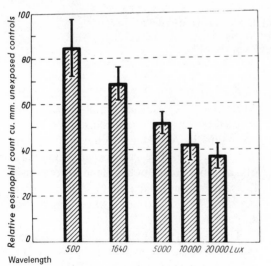

Wavelength

Fig. 31. Mean relative eosinophil counts in female mice of uniform age 60 minutes after a one-hour period of exposure to white artificial light at various levels of intensity.

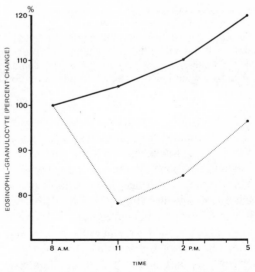

Fig. 33. Diurnal variation in 300 blind and 50 normal-sighted individuals. In the normal sighted there is a significant fall in the value of eosinophils in the forenoon which is missing in the blind. Dotted line, normal sighted (n = 50); solid line, blind (n = 300).

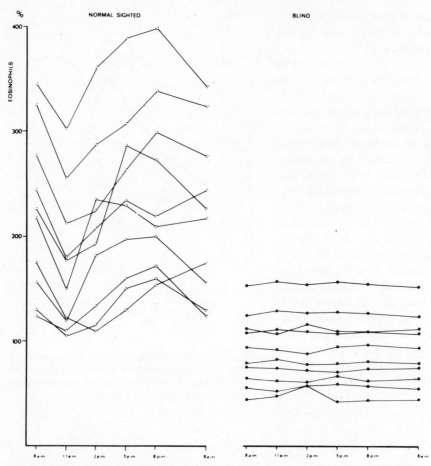

Fig. 34. Circadian eosinophil rhythm (individual curves) in both the blind and persons with normal ocular light perception. Individual pattern of the diurnal fluctuation of eosinophils in the two categories. Diminution of the diurnal rhythm in the blind with a reduction of the total number of eosinophils in the blood.

1973, 1974), the presence of a sinusoid eosinophil movement corresponding to the physiological light-darkness rhythm was established in persons with normal sight (Fig. 32). This rhythm is no longer ascertainable in 300 blind test subjects (Figs. 33, 34). If the behavior of eosinophilic movement is observed in patients blinded by cataracts before and after removal of the opaque lens, then preoperatively only a faint or virtually nonexistent eosinophil drop can be traced; postoperatively, however, normal physiological behavior is restored (Fig. 35). Totally blind test subjects who demonstrated neither matutinal eosinopenia nor the diurnal sinusoid pattern reacted to intramuscular ACTH in-

jections with a sudden fall in eosinophils, which indicates normal functioning of the adrenal cortex but at the same time an abnormality in ACTH excretion by the pituitary (Fig. 36). The postoperative influence of light on cataract patients therefore causes the same eosinopenic effect as the preoperative ACTH injections when light was excluded.

This becomes especially clear in comparing the behavior of eosinophils when ACTH is injected with the reaction to light stress in the form of flicker light treatment: after adaptation to darkness intermittent photostimuli elicit marked eosinopenia, which, according to Radnot and Wallner (1965), can

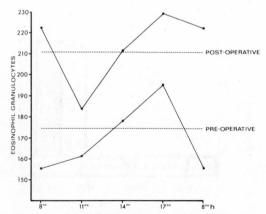

Fig. 35. Behavior of eosinophils before and after cataract extraction (n = 50). The chart shows the change of eosinophils of 50 cataract patients with a vision less than 1/20. There is an absence of the normal morning eosinopenia in the blind. After cataract extraction restoration of normal behavior (morning fall of eosinophils) occurs in the same subjects.

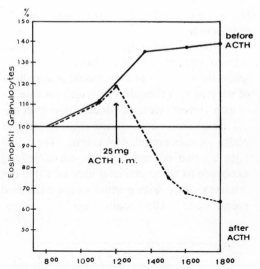

Fig. 36. Thorn-Test of 25 practically blind cataract patients. There is no decrease of eosinophils in the morning in blind patients. The same patients show an eosinopenia of 52 percent after the injection of ACTH. This confirms that the adrenal glands in cataract-blinded patients are well functioning. The reason for the absence of morning eosinopenia is therefore the lack of light induction of the adrenal glands by the way of the hypothalamic-hypophyseal system.

be used to test retina function in the case of opaque media. A significant dependence of eosinopenia on vision was noted: with 1/20 vision eosinopenia did not occur, with 1/10 it appeared beneath the physiological threshold, with 1/5 it began to approach normal values (Fig. 37).

Halberg and Vissher (1950) conducted research on the behavior of eosinophils in nocturnal laboratory animals. Inbred strains of mice exhibited lower eosinophil values at midnight than in the morning. In further experiments Halberg et al (1953a) investigated the influence of feeding, social stimuli, and environmental conditions in addition to the effect of constant light. If the rhythm of exposure to light was reversed, eosinophil values also showed an inversion after an interval of four to five days. A change in feeding times and the use of food with reduced caloric content produced the same effect, although more slowly. Rats also showed lower eosinophil values at night than in the morning (Halberg et al 1954a). In blind as well as enucleated mice (Halberg et al 1954b), diurnal and nocturnal values proved to be similar after enucleation and after the exclusion of light. In cases of blindness from

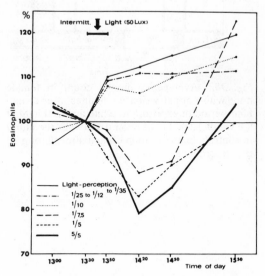

Fig. 37. Fifty cataract patients with different visual acuity were exposed to intermittent flicker light (intensity of illumination 50 lux, 60 flashes per minute; light-darkness ratio 1:1). With weak visual acuity (reduced light perception) the eosinopenic effect of the light is weak; when visual acuity increases (more light perception), the effect is stronger.

birth, environmental factors alone are of importance.

Hollwich and Tilgner (1963b) exposed normal sighted and blind mice to artificial white light as well as to monochromatic light of varying wavelengths. Two different series of experiments were conducted under identical conditions and during the ascendant phase of eosinophil movement. They discovered that 60 minutes after an hour-long exposure to white artificial light of 1,000 lux intensity, mice with normal vision exhibited pronounced, statistically verified eosin-

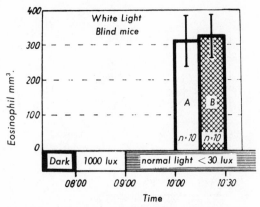

Fig. 39. Average eosinophil count in blind mice 60 minutes after a one-hour period of exposure to white artificial light (1,000 lux). Group A is compared with the count in blind controls (Group B).

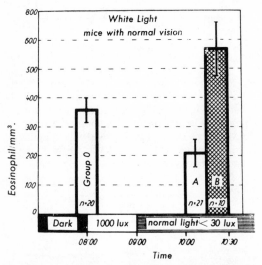

Fig. 38. Average eosinophil count in female mice with normal vision 60 minutes after a one-hour period of exposure to white artificial light at a level of 1,000 lux (A) compared with the count in controls before (Group O) and after (Group B) the experiment.

openia of about 36 percent (Fig. 38). Under identical experimental conditions, blind animals on the other hand did not display eosinopenia (Fig. 39). The exposure to different wavelengths (436, 546, 632, and 707 nm) resulted in an eosinopenia of 65-70 percent. These experiments demonstrate that intensive exposure of the eyes to light apparently lowers the eosinophil count by increasing the activity of the adrenal cortex.

In the mouse there is a quantitative, linear relationship between the logarithm of the intensity of exposure and the magnitude of the eosinopenic effect (Tilgner 1966, 1967). To summarize, these findings reveal that in animals as well as humans the occurrence of eosinopenia caused by photostimulus is linked to the ocular perception of light.

8

Light and Metabolic Functions

Endogenic Lipid Metabolism

Until approximately 1926 research in the field of internal medicine appeared to indicate that the concentration of serum cholesterol is virtually constant in the healthy person insofar as alimentary stress does not cause an increase which then disappears after a few hours. A series of experiments conducted by Georgi (1944) demonstrated that blood samples taken at the same time of day from males in good mental and physical health did not reveal any significant fluctuations in serum cholesterol over a period of weeks and months. In contrast to the mentally healthy, the mentally ill suffering from depression showed increased cholesterol levels ranging from slight to severe. In order better to understand this abnormality in cholesterol balance, Georgi conducted cholesterol tolerance tests (using olive oil) finding that the levels of blood cholesterol produced a curve. He searched subsequently for autonomic fluctuations in concentration that were not induced by stress and discovered a diurnal curve with a rise in the morning, a peak at noon, and a drop in the afternoon.

Peterson et al (1960) divided their test persons (healthy medical students) into so-called labile subjects and stabile subjects following lengthy preliminary tests to determine the constancy of their cholesterol content. The test subjects were brought to an emotionally agitated state by means of sophisticated methods of stimulation (cold, acoustical stimuli, psychic stress), and then their cholesterol fluctuations were compared. Without stress, a diurnal rhythm was found with a matutinal rise, a midday drop, and a sharp rise in the evening, which then dropped again at night. With additional psychic stress, however, the labile group exhibited considerable deviations in their cholesterol fluctuations.

Stöckli (1966) attempted to refine these findings by studying 15 nonhospitalized people with normal metabolism. He discovered rhythmic diurnal cholesterol fluctuations of a regular nature in these experimental subjects. Among them were some individuals with slight and some with considerable fluctuations. His curves revealed also a consistent matutinal rise reaching a midday peak with a subsequent marked cholesterol drop ending during the course of the afternoon.

Using 48 subjects, Buhl (1966) conducted

a series of tests which extended into the night as well. He found varying curves which he divided into six main groups. Common to them all was a basic four-hour rhythm, interrupted by a three-, five-, or seven-hour rhythm around the time of midday and afternoon. In all these groups, in the afternoon and evening as well as in the night there was a cholesterol drop which showed a tendency to approach the matutinal (fasting) level.

The extent of endogenic cholesterol biosynthesis, a function of the liver, depends principally on the cholesterol content of the diet, since cholesterol has an inhibitory effect on its own biosynthesis. On the other hand, along with the carbohydrate and fat content of the diet, numerous hormones affect cholesterol metabolism: insulin deficiency increases synthesis and blood levels; the thyroid hormone and estrogen have an antagonistic effect.

It is not only cholesterol that exhibits an endogenic rhythm. In comparative experiments with normal sighted and enucleated rats under natural conditions of light and darkness, Hollwich et al (1966) demonstrated in the rats with normal sight a 60 percent increase in free fatty acids paralleling an increase in daylight, whereas enucleated rats under the same conditions of light, heat, and diet did not reveal any changes in the free fatty acids in their serum—neither did the control animals kept in darkness. Similar experiments on rabbits who had been subjected to a five-day-long period of darkness preceding the test showed comparable results. Hollwich et al (1966) studied further the effect of light stress on the metabolism of free fatty acids, attempting to determine to what degree the effect of stress-inducing photostimuli on fat metabolism proceeds via the eye. Exposed to flicker light as well as to regular light, animals with normal sight displayed an increase in free fatty acids. In rats and rabbits, normal daylight and artificial light affect fat metabolism by increasing the free fatty acids in the serum; these effects depend, however, on intact ocular perception of light.

The first studies of fat metabolism in the blind were made by Hollwich and Dieckhues (1967c). Twenty-five cataract patients whose blood was taken under identical conditions before surgery showed an elevation in serum cholesterol and free fatty acids which receded to normal levels after surgery when the influence of light had been restored. Another study showed that persons with impaired vision demonstrated a fat metabolism behavior located between that of the blind and normal sighted (Hollwich and Dieckhues 1971b,c). Plasma concentration of free fatty acids is regulated by a large number of nutritive and nervous factors. But here, too, the hormones that are dependent on the diencephalic-pituitary system—adrenalin, somatotropic hormone (STH),* ACTH, thyrotropin (TSH),† thyroid, and corticosteroids—again appear as direct or indirect lipolytic factors. Thus, the connection with "the energetic portion of the optic pathway" is once again established.

Protein Metabolism

Farkas (1928) described a rhythm in the component parts of blood plasma. He found a certain regularity in the shift of protein fractions in favor of globulins. Total protein decreased toward evening. These findings were tested and confirmed by Lang (1930). In 15 out of 20 cases he discovered a globulin increase toward evening. Only three cases showed no fluctuation and two showed an increase in albumen. By continuously measuring serum proteins over a period of several days, Döring et al (1951) discovered a pronounced diurnal rhythm with a minimum in the early morning hours. When the sleep-waking rhythm was reversed, they observed a shift in the protein minimum along with the altered sleep pattern. The results of a further series of measurements conducted on exper-

*Peptide hormone of the pituitary gland. Influences growth and fat and glucose metabolism (diabetogenic effect). Also known as human growth hormone (HGH).
†Thyroid stimulating hormone.

imental subjects confined to bed deviate in amplitude but not in rhythm from the results of the series conducted on experimental subjects following a normal sleep and work rhythm. Based on their comparative observations of the three series of tests, the authors concluded that diurnal fluctuations in serum protein content are related to the sleep rhythm; the alternation between muscular activity and rest causes an increase in normal fluctuation. In addition, they discuss the influence of the tumefaction of proteins and of "hydremia," brought about by the stronger effect of the antidiuretic hormone at night.

At present there are no data on the diurnal rhythm of blood protein content in the blind. Hollwich and Dieckhues (1971b,c) did find a change in protein metabolism in the blind in the form of a negative nitrogen balance accompanied by increased protein metabolism (lowered serum protein values, a rise in rest nitrogen, uric acid, and creatinine in the serum). In cataract patients the nitrogen balance (rise in serum protein) became normal after surgery.

Liver Metabolism

Forsgren (1935) studied in detail the liver's role as the central controlling organ for intermediary metabolism. Along with its dominant role in carbohydrate metabolism, the liver also performs important tasks in amino acid and nitrogen metabolism, in serum protein synthesis, lipid metabolism, enzyme synthesis, detoxification, and choleresis. It would be too time consuming to describe all the specific regulatory mechanisms and diurnal rhythms, but those metabolic activities dependent on light should be mentioned.

The detoxifying role of the liver may be taken as a criterion for hepatic function in animal experiments. Reid-Hunt (1905) introduced acetonitrile lethality in mice as a reproducible experimental model. The actual toxic effect seems to stem from prussic acid released over a long period. The disappearance of this reaction was explained by sea-

sonal and nutritionally determined fluctuations in thyroid activity.

Santo (1934), however, demonstrated that there was not a direct parallel between acetonitrile lethality and thyroid activity and established that daylight or darkness alters the outcome of the experiment, but he did not find accompanying histological changes in the thyroid gland. Light had the effect of heightening resistance.

Proceeding from these experiments, Hollwich and Dieckhues (1966) tested the sensitivity of white mice to acetonitrile under normal and abnormal diurnal rhythms in light-darkness conditions (Fig. 40). Further series of experiments with normal sighted and enucleated mice dealt with the influence of constant light as well as of diurnal periodicity on lethality. Lethality increased signifi-

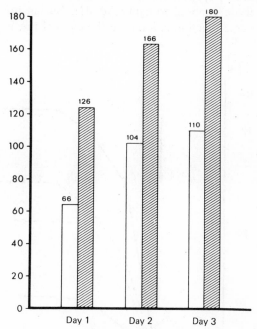

Fig. 40. Acetonitrile lethality (500 white mice). Of 500 white mice, 250 were kept in the light and 250 in darkness. After five days each mouse was injected subcutaneously with 1 mg of acetonitrile per g body weight. After one day, 66 of the animals kept in the light and 126 of those kept in darkness died. Three days after the injection the lethality ratio was 110 of the animals in light to 180 of the animals in darkness. Open bar, light; hatched bar, darkness.

cantly when light perception via the "energetic portion" of the optic pathway was eliminated by darkness or enucleation. A disturbance of the light-darkness rhythm also influenced sensitivity to acetonitrile, depending on the duration of the disturbance. Furthermore there were fluctuations in toxicity according to the time of day, with the lowest degree of lethality occurring during the afternoon when the experimental animals had been exposed to daylight for eight hours.

Later experiments (Hollwich and Dieckhues 1974a) involved the injection of two substances with differing effects: on the one hand Nembutal, which is broken down by the liver into nontoxic products, on the other hand a primarily nontoxic substance (E 605), which the liver transformed into a toxic compound. Nembutal lethality among the mice kept in darkness was greater than in those exposed to light (Fig. 41). But an inverse reaction is found in the case of the E 605 injection. The reason for this lies in the differing toxic effects of the two chemical substances: whereas Nembutal is detoxified in the liver, E 605 (nitrostigmin) is transformed by the liver's metabolic action into the toxic cholinesterase mintacol. Since the breakdown of Nembutal and the transformation of E 605 take place primarily in the liver, it can be concluded from these experiments that there is reduced liver metabolism in the animals kept in darkness.

Hecht et al (1968) report on a series of pharmacological effects dependent on the brightness of the environment; they point out the significance of their findings for pharmacological and pharmaceutical research as well as for pharmacotherapy with humans. Nelson and Halberg (1973) investigated circadian rhythm in the sleep response of mice injected with different doses of pentobarbital. Significant differences were found at different times of day in the length of sleep as well as in the animals' plasma level.

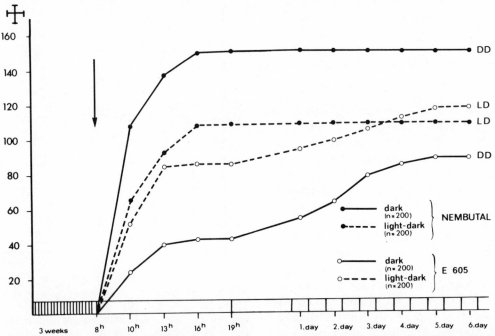

Fig. 41. Nembutal and E 605 lethality of white mice in light and in darkness. For the mice kept in darkness lethality after injection of Nembutal is greater than in the animals in light (breakdown of toxic Nembutal by the liver). On the other hand, with the injection of E 605 lethality among the mice in darkness is less than among those in light (transformation by the liver of primarily nontoxic E 605 into a compound with toxic effect).

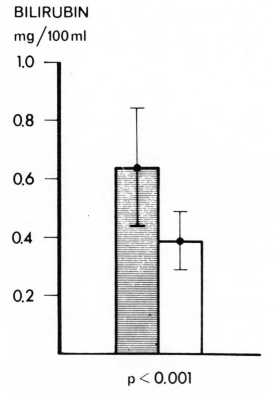

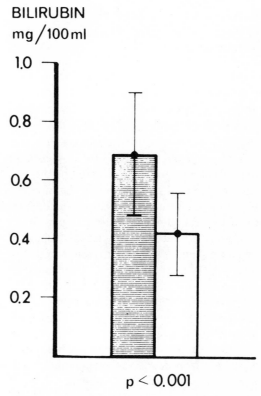

Fig. 42A. Bilirubin content in the serum of the blind compared to those with sight. In the blind there is a significant rise in the bilirubin level in the serum. Hatched bar, blind (n = 400); open bar, normal sighted (n = 80).

Fig. 42B. Bilirubin content in the serum of cataract patients before (blind) and after (vision restored) cataract operation. The increased bilirubin content of the serum before surgery becomes normal as a result of the restored ocular perception of light. Hatched bar, before surgery, (n = 150); open bar, after surgery.

Cremer et al (1958) demonstrated the practical application of a photochemical phenomenon when bilirubin is broken down by light: blue fluorescent light caused a reduction of bilirubin in the serum of the newborn. Friederiszick and Seitz (1970) reported on the clinical results of phototherapy based on the use of this light in the treatment of icterus in the newborn. Sisson (1973) compared the effectiveness in the therapy of jaundice in the newborn (premature and full-term births), but he tested only the treatment of existing hyperbilirubinemia and not its prophylaxis. Phototherapy proved to be a very effective method of treatment, regardless of whether premature or full-term births were involved.

Hollwich and Dieckhues (1974a) investigated the influence of light on the liver's bilirubin metabolism in both the blind and normal sighted (Fig. 42A, B). Bilirubin, which originates as hemoglobin, is broken down in the reticuloendothelial system, is not water soluble, and thus cannot be urinated. In one of the liver's typical metabolic functions it is conjugated into water soluble bilirubin-glucoronid and eliminated into the intestine via the biliary ducts. Comparative examination of the blind and normal sighted reveals that the bilirubin level in the serum of the blind is significantly higher than in the normal sighted. One hundred and fifty patients with cataracts who were virtually blind also displayed the stimulatory effect of light on liver metabolism. Whereas an increased bilirubin content was found before surgery, it became normal after surgery, i.e., after unimpeded entry of light into the eye had been restored.

Carbohydrate Balance

Experimental and clinical observations have shown consistently that the diencephalon can play a regulatory role in almost all autonomically controlled processes of the organism. Isolated deficiencies in this area of the brain must thus lead to abnormalities in regulatory functions in the total organism.

Claude Bernard (1885) with his "diabetic puncture" and Bouchardat (1851) with his discovery of the pathogenetic significance of the pancreas for diabetes did the first scientific research in this field. Langerhans (1869) was the first to establish that carbohydrate metabolism is regulated by the islet of the pancreas. In 1889 Mehring and Minkowski were able to produce diabetes mellitus in a dog by means of pancreatectomy.

Since that time experiments and clinical observations have consistently demonstrated that mutual cooperation between the pituitary and diencephalon is a significant element in the regulation of metabolic processes. This is also true for sugar metabolism, for the data found in the literature reveal that there is almost certainly a close connection between carbohydrate balance and the diencephalon.

For example, Dubois (1902) described a "center" in the wall of the third ventricle that when stimulated in laboratory animals produced a decrease in glycogen formation in the liver as well as induced sleep and altered the rhythm of breathing. Aschner (1929) showed that "by puncturing the base of the 3rd ventricle, glycosuria of up to 4 percent and lasting 1 to 2 days can be produced." This operation, which Aschner called a "hypothalamic diabetic puncture," is completely successful, that is, it leads to hyperglycemia and glycosuria even after total extirpation of the anterior and posterior lobes of the pituitary. It is just as successful even after the third ventricle is damaged

from above, in other words, when there is careful avoidance of injury to the pituitary.

These experimental findings were corroborated by Leschke (1918) as well as by Camus and Roussy (1920). In experiments with rabbits with an injured tuber cinereum, Camus et al (1923) always observed the occurrence of diabetes with glycemia if the tuber nuclei and the nucleus paraventricularis were injured. Himwich and Keller (1933) found that direct stimulation of the hypothalamus resulted in hyperglycemia; D'Amour and Keller (1933) were able to cause hypoglycemic conditions by operating on the anterior hypothalamus. After cauterizing the hypothalamus of dogs with silver nitrate, Strieck (1937) produced diabetes mellitus with hyperglycemia of 200 mg percent, which remained constant until the animal's death, and with glycosuria of three percent without an increase in basal metabolism or alterations in temperature, pulse, or breathing. The pathological-anatomical control indicated extensive necrosis in the hypothalamic region.

Barris and Ingram (1936) injured the hypothalamus in cats, producing temporary hyperglycemia with glycosuria. In those cases in which the nucleus paraventricularis was destroyed, permanent hypoglycemia followed the temporary hypoglycemia, and in addition an extreme sensitivity to insulin developed.

The findings of Morgan et al (1937) agree with these experimental observations concerning the close connection between the hypothalamus and pancreas; in five cases of diabetes mellitus, they found considerable cell reduction and cell loss in the nucleus paraventricularis. Thus, these authors describe the nucleus paraventricularis as the central stimulator of pancreas function, in other words, as a "sugar center."

Blood Sugar

Numerous studies attest to the fact that light induces carbohydrate metabolism. Diurnal fluctuations in carbohydrate metabolism

which are related to the periodic change between light and darkness can be observed.

Moleschott (1855) thought he could prove
that animals in light produce more carbonic
acid than they do in darkness. Blind animals
also were supposed to produce less carbon
dioxide in darkness than in the light. Graffenberger's research (1893) proceeded from
the fact that agricultural animals are easier
to fatten in dark places than when they are
kept in very bright areas. He discovered that
the withdrawal of light caused production of
more body fat, without however having any
effect on the synthesis of liver glycogen. The
first finding became a well known fact, the
second can probably be attributed to the
inadequate research methods of that time.

Gigon (1929) cleared up this matter by
keeping healthy rabbits in complete darkness and then testing their blood sugar level
after glucose and levulose tolerance tests.
When he compared the nitrogen and carbon
content of the blood, it became clear that the
absence of light led to an abnormality in
sugar assimilation, which proceeded normally only in the presence of light.

Jores (1934) found that blood sugar levels
were higher in four rabbits whose eyes were
kept closed by clamps for three days than in
animals who had been kept in the normal
diurnal rhythms of light and darkness. More
recent experiments (Hollwich and Dieckhues 1967b) confirm Jores' findings: after
light's entry into the eyes has been eliminated, there is first of all a rise in blood sugar
until the fourth day, followed by an abrupt
and then a later gradual fall to subnormal
hypoglycemic levels (Fig. 43).

Forsgren (1935) found a diurnally
rhythmic fluctuation in liver glycogen in experiments with rabbits and on this basis associated human carbohydrate metabolism
with the liver. Deuel et al (1938) made the
same observation in rats.

In detailed metabolic experiments with
chicks, Elfvin et al (1955) traced the course
of the diurnal curve of liver glycogen. Given
the normal physiological light-darkness alternation, liver glycogen exhibits a 24-hour
rhythm with a nocturnal minimum. The

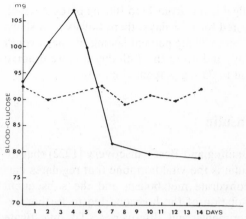

Fig. 43. Influence of darkness on the blood/
glucose level. Blood sugar was measured daily at
8:30 A.M. on an empty stomach in 25 patients
experiencing total darkness. After an initial sharp
rise up to the fourth day, there followed a drop in
blood sugar to subnormal values, at first sharp
and later more gradual. The fasting value of blood
sugar in the normal sighted, on the other hand,
shows only slight fluctuations. Solid line, 25 people binocular; broken line, 25 people in normal
light-dark rhythm.

change from dissimilation to assimilation
(called the intermediary phase by these authors) takes place during the night. An inverse light-darkness rhythm causes an inversion of the glycogen rhythm—the length of
the intermediary phase is proportional to
that of the period of darkness. In these authors' opinion this diurnal biorhythm is influenced by exogenic factors (among them
the earth's rotation, day-night change in
light intensity, temperature, and so on) and
endogenic ones (autonomic nervous system
and hormones). Halberg et al (1960) discovered a similar situation in their experiments
on mice.

Raab (1939) noted a fall in blood sugar
levels after a seven-, nine-, or fifteen-day
confinement to darkness undergone by five
human volunteers wearing bandages over
both eyes.

Hollwich and Dieckhues (1967b) conducted similar experiments on 25 patients
with eye ailments who wore bandages over
both eyes. In agreement with Jores' findings,
they first observed an increase in blood

sugar levels from 93 to 106 mg percent which lasted for four days, then, however, a sharp drop to 83 mg percent lasting till the seventh day, and up to the 14th day a more gradual fall to 75 mg percent (Fig. 43).

Insulin

Banting and Best's discovery (1922) that insulin is the vital hormone that regulates carbohydrate metabolism and the subsequent isolation of the hormone led to further experiments and discoveries. To investigate the question of whether or in what way the absence of photo impulses affects the regulation of carbohydrate metabolism, we (Hollwich et al.) included grape sugar and insulin tolerance tests in the experiments.

As early as 1950, Hollwich had conducted a *functional test of carbohydrate balance* on blind subjects based on a method developed by Staub and Traugott. This method involves a double alimentary glucose tolerance test administered with an interval of one and one-half hours. In the healthy person the second dose of grape sugar, which is

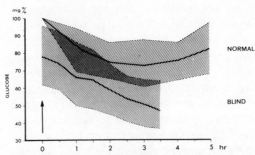

Fig. 44.   Average curve of the blood-sugar level of 40 persons born blind compared with normal-sighted persons after insulin test (Radoslav) with subcutaneous injection of 0.2 E/kg body weight.

given at the time when the blood sugar is normally already falling, either causes no rise in blood sugar at all or only a slight additional one.

In his first orientative experiments on ten blind persons and using Staub and Traugott's double grape sugar tolerance test, Hollwich obtained negative results seven times in the form of a deviation from the norm. Only three times did he find a normal reaction. In these cases of initial reduced reactivity, the rise in blood sugar after the

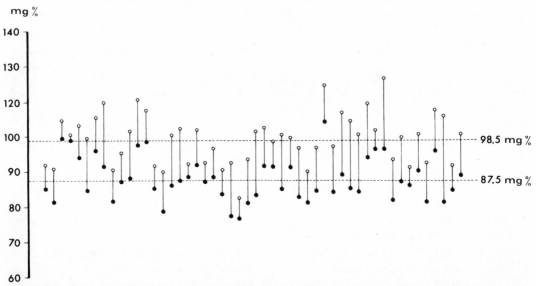

Fig. 45.   Behavior of blood sugar of 25 patients before and after cataract surgery. After the vision has been reestablished the average value of blood sugar increases from 85.6 mg% to 98.5 mg%. Closed circle, before surgery; open circle, after surgery.

first tolerance test was lower than the norm whereas after the second test it always exceeded the first peak. Thus, Hollwich found in the blind a reaction deviating from the norm both in the first and the second rise in blood sugar. His findings were corroborated by Fuchs (1953), von Schumann (1953), and Wassner (1954). In the following years, Hollwich validated his findings through the use of increased numbers of patients (Hollwich 1963; Hollwich and Dieckhues 1967).

The *insulin tolerance test based on Radoslav* (Hollwich 1954, 1965) is used today especially in cases of abnormality in STH secretion. In those persons with normal metabolism, it causes a drop in blood sugar to half of the original level after half an hour and a simultaneous sharp, long-lasting rise in STH in the blood. As a result of the pituitary's counter-regulatory action, the original level is reached again or is exceeded after one to one and one-half hours. In blind persons to whom the insulin tolerance test is administered blood sugar drops far below the critical level, which indicates that the pituitary's antagonistic counter-regulation takes place only belatedly and below the physiological threshold (Fig. 44). Thus, according to Hollwich, the results of both tolerance tests indicate a connection between blindness and a dysfunction of the hypophysial portion of blood sugar regulation.

If the behavior of blood sugar in *cataract patients* is tested *before and after surgery* (Hollwich and Dieckhues, 1967b, 1971a,b,c), a significant rise in blood sugar from 87.5 mg percent to 98.5 mg percent is found after surgery under unchanging conditions of diet and environment (Fig. 45). The varying results of the Staub-Traugott tolerance test seen in the virtually blind state before surgery and in the state of restored sight after surgery can, under the same unvariable and stationary environmental conditions, serve as a further proof that light's entry into the eye has an influence on the regulation of sugar balance (Fig. 46).

In recent times, several researchers have described a diurnal rhythm of insulin secretion, which has become measurable by

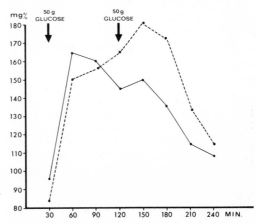

Fig. 46. Glucose stress (Staub-Traugott) of 25 patients before and after cataract surgery. Fifty g of glucose was given to 25 "blinded" cataract patients, and again 50 g after one and one-half hours. The blood sugar was determined every half-hour. After the second administration the increase of blood sugar was much higher than after the first one creating the two-peaked curve with an enlarged second peak. After vision had been reestablished the second blood sugar peak was smaller because of sufficient production of insulin. Solid line, before surgery; broken line, after surgery.

means of exact quantitative radioimmunological methods (Jarrett 1974; Lakatua et al 1974a,b; Lestradet et al 1974; Reinberg et al 1974; Thum et al 1975). On the basis of previous knowledge, insulin secretion was assumed to interfere with the cortisone and STH rhythms (Lestradet 1974; Lakatua et al 1974). The continuing study of the diurnal profile of blood sugar in correlation with serum insulin (Thum et al 1975) in particular provides the possibility of assessing precisely light's effect on carbohydrate metabolism by means of future light experiments with normal sighted and blind subjects. In view of today's knowledge, the constancy of this metabolic rhythm and the preservation of normal levels are maintained by two interrelated regulatory systems: 1) alimentary regulation of blood sugar performed principally by the hormones of the pancreas and the adrenal glands; and 2) central autonomic regulation which is influenced by light's entry into the eye and is controlled by the diencephalic-pituitary system.

9

Light and Thyroid Function

The close connection between the functions of the gonads and the thyroid in their effect on growth, reproduction, molting, and bird migration prompted experiments concerning the influence of varying light conditions on thyroid function. Schildmacher (1938) discovered that the thyroid colloid of the male garden redstart evidenced absorption in the fall (September to December). The degree of absorption was not noticeably influenced by additional exposure to light or the injection of male sex hormones. On the other hand, the injection of thyroxine was very effective; thyroid glands in a storage state with an extremely flat epithelium were formed. Exposure to artificially lengthened days from March to April caused molting and weight increase in castrated male green finches; the thyroid's advanced state of absorption indicates the organ's heightened activity (Rautenberg 1952). Artificially shortened days in summer do not affect the annual rhythm of thyroid activity in green finches. Exposure to lengthened days, however, increases the production of the thyrotropic (TSH) hormone (Schildmacher 1956).

In the fall season, Tixier-Vidal and As-senmacher (1959) studied seven-month-old male Peking ducks who had been raised in a natural environment and were in a condition of autumnal gonad involution. Under constant temperature conditions, they were exposed either to constant light or constant darkness for three weeks in order to test the effect of varying light conditions on thyroid function. In a control group kept in natural light conditions, moderately heightened thyroid excretion appeared with simultaneously heightened iodine fixation and sharply increased synthesis and storage. Constant light effected additional stimulation of thyroid function, constant darkness brought about a reduction. The most pronounced period of thyroid function when testicular development begins in the months of January and February is followed by a drop in activity as the testes approach their maximum functioning (March and April).

Hollwich and Tilgner (1962) expanded upon the experiments by Benoit (1934, 1938, 1961a,b, 1964) and Tixier-Vidal and Assenmacher (1959) involving photostimulation of the gonads. They studied 95 Peking ducks over a period of five years. The thyroid was also studied in order to trace the connections between gonad development and thyroid function (Fig. 47). Among the various possible ways of obtaining information on thyroid activity, the authors chose to measure the size of the cell nucleus. Irradiation of the ocular regions of five-month-old drakes with monochromatic light having a wavelength of 707 nm (red light) resulted in an increased average volume of the cell nuclei of the follicles; this was an expression of an increase in functional activity. Here for the first time a connection was established experimentally between the wavelength of the light entering the eye and the size of the nuclei found in the thyroid. The differences in the volumes of the follicle cell nuclei may to a certain extent be considered the expression of functional or metabolic changes in the thyroid. Radnot and Orban (1955), working with ducks, also obtained results pointing to a stimulating influence of light on the thyroid.

Bergfeld (1930) attributed the seasonal differences in thyroid activity in rabbits to the seasonal variations in light intensity. Santo (1934) tested the effect of light on acetonitrile resistance in white mice. Animals with a heightened thyroid activity that were kept in darkness required lower doses to cause death, animals kept in light needed higher doses. Brands (1954) found that light causes a significant drop in stored radioactive iodine in the thyroid of mice. Miline (1952) irradiated the eyes of adult rabbits while shielding their bodies from the light. White light caused a fall in thyroid activity, while red light caused a rise. Milin and Ciglar (1956) observed histological signs of thyroid hyperfunction in rabbits after irradiation with sunlight.

Constant light as well as constant darkness affects thyroid activity in white mice (Puntriano and Meites 1951). In constant light there is a marked reduction in thyroid weight, radioactive iodine absorption, and thiouracil reaction; on the other hand, in constant darkness these increase. It appears that constant light results in reduced thyroid

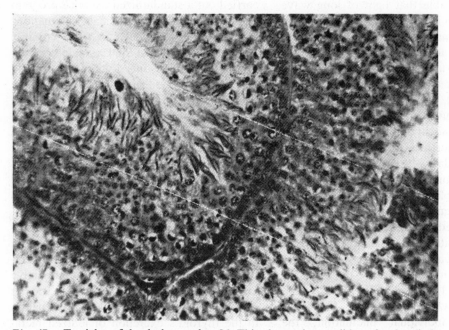

Fig. 47.   Testicles of the drake number 86. This shows the condition after irradiation of the ocular region with monochromatic light with a wavelength of 707 nm (intensity of illumination 2.45 × 10^{-4}W/cm²; total duration of illumination 120 hours within 29 days). Uninterrupted stages of spermatocystogenesis and spermiohistogenesis. Chromium-osmium-acetic acid. Paraffin 6. Scale, 250:1.

function in mice, while constant darkness results in increased function. Dale et al (1972) exposed growing rabbits to varying periods of light and then measured the content of iodized amino acids in their thyroid and the TSH content of the pituitary. The group of rabbits in constant light showed the greatest increase in thyroid synthesis and TSH content, the reverse effect was found for the group in constant darkness. In the opinion of Dale et al, these results indicate clearly that constant light stimulates the hypothalamic-pituitary-thyroid axis. Shimada et al (1973) recorded the EEG of the hypothalamus in chickens stimulated by flicker light. The EEG waves of the tested region were directly related to flicker frequency. The authors were able to prove that, depending on flicker frequency, protein-bound iodine (PBI)* rose significantly as a parameter for the amount of thyroid hormone in the serum.

All these observations point to light's thyrotropic effect, although the question of how this comes about remains open at present. It is highly probable that light of long wave length plays an important role here, as in the case of the gonads.

Walfish et al (1961) suspected diurnally rhythmic fluctuations of the thyroid hormones in humans when they discovered fluctuations in the serum of persons with euthyroidism after a single injection of radioactively marked thyroxine. The rate of disappearance increases progressively in the course of the day, reaching a maximum at 2 A.M. The authors attribute this phenomenon to changes in plasma volume. Studies of the dynamics of endogenic iodine metabolism were conducted by Mertz and Isele (1964). They investigated the dynamics of thyroid function by measuring the serum concentration of PBI for two to three days after a tracer dose had been administered to young healthy males with euthyroidism. In spite of considerable individual fluctuation, the mean values of PBI concentration in the serum are lowest in the morning hours,

reaching a maximum at midnight; the differences in mean value between the midnight maximum and matutinal minimum are statistically significant here. Total iodine-131 concentration in the serum displays a similar 24-hour characteristic pattern. The authors exclude the possibility of a "thinning effect" of plasma as the cause of the diurnally periodic fluctuations, leaving unanswered the question of whether a central phenomenon at the level of the hypothalamus is involved in the dynamics of iodine metabolism or whether peripheral interferences with other factors play a role.

Motivated by the partially equivocal findings on the diurnal rhythm of thyroid hormones, Vernikos-Danellis et al (1972) undertook a long-term study of eight healthy hospitalized males in whom the disturbing influences of their customary environment and activity rhythms were eliminated. During the eight weeks that the experiment lasted, serum concentration of the thyroid hormones was measured repeatedly over periods of 48 hours. Half of the test subjects carried out a standardized exercise program in bed. There were significant fluctuations for T3 (triiodotyronine) and T4 (thyroxin)* with the maximum at 7:30 A.M. In contrast to the stable cortisone rhythm, the thyroid hormones exhibited an essentially less stable diurnal rhythm, which did however return completely to its regular phasic condition upon increased bed rest, particularly in the subsequent ten-day control period. These authors suspect that thyroid rhythm is dependent on body position. De Costre et al (1971) also reported that the serum T4 values reached a maximum between 8 A.M. and 1 P.M. and a minimum at 2 A.M. They attributed these variations to hydremia along with changes in position during the night. Nicoloff (1970) measured variations in radioactive iodine excreted in the urine. In this way he also found a diurnally rhythmic fluctuation in the thyroid's excretion of iodized metabolic products. His measurements still

---

*Total iodine bound to protein in the thyroid gland.

*Hormones are secreted by the thyroid gland and influence basal metabolism by increasing oxidation (mitochondria).

pointed, however, to an inverse rhythm—a maximum between 40 minutes after midnight and 7:20 A.M. and a minimum between 1:20 P.M. and 8:40 P.M.—in other words, high levels of excretion during the period of minimal activity.

O'Connor et al (1974) applied radioimmunological methods to trace the plasma-thyroxine profile in healthy males. They measured the plasma concentration of T4 at 20-minute intervals; with the use of this short-interval collection technique, they demonstrated the existence of sudden, short-term T4 fluctuations in all the test subjects. The average T4 concentration was slightly higher during the waking period than during sleep—in other words, relatively constant in general. O'Connor et al were not certain that the rises in T4 concentration are of thyroidal nature. Studies of the diurnal fluctuations of TSH can be illuminating here but have thus far often yielded unsatisfactory results (Vanhaelst et al 1972; Webster et al 1972; Weeke 1973).

Hollwich (1973, 1974) was the first to report on studies of thyroid function in the blind. He measured the free capacity of the thyroxine-binding protein (T3 test) as well as serum thyroxine (T4 test) as parameters for thyroid activity. A slight but significant thyroid hypofunction was found in the blind as compared to healthy control subjects. The same observation was made when comparing the condition of cataract patients before and after surgery. Serum thyroxine became normal when the entry of light into the eye was restored; the T3 test remained unchanged. His co-worker Dieckhues (1974) expanded the experiments to include the measurement of diurnal hormone curves. Amplitude is reduced in the blind and mean values are lower than for the normal sighted. Here too, the comparison of individual curves for the blind and normal sighted impressively demonstrates differences in the fluctuations in the diurnal hormone curves caused by the absence of light's stimulatory and regulatory effect as it enters the eye.

10
Light and Sexual Function

It has long been suspected that light conditions play a role in the annual cycle of the sexual function in animals. Rowan (1925–1928), for example, observed North American finches who migrate every fall to their far distant winter quarters in the south. In captured birds, artificial daylight approximating the length of days in summer induced premature activity of the gonads, which had already regressed to their winter minimum. This exposure to light interrupted the natural migratory rhythm. Upon being set free, the finches broke off their migration and returned north even though it was still winter.

Rowan concluded from this that scarcity of food and weather conditions are only external motives for bird migration. In his view, the annual flight of the finches he studied depends on two factors: the inner physiological factor of the gonads, which, during a certain stage of development and activity, is regulated by an external factor, the length of daylight.

Bissonette (1931, 1932, 1933, 1939) studied the sexual function in starlings and jays. By exposing the birds to red light at night, he succeeded in shortening the period of winter dormancy of their gonads. The acceleration of gonadal development and spermatogenesis proceeded in proportion to the degree of increase in light intensity. Full spermatogenesis and activation of the epididymus, which usually do not occur until brooding time, now took place in December.

Ringeon (1942) observed the effects of extended exposure to red or green light in the house sparrow. By means of red light he induced an almost full maturation of the gonads in the female as well as male birds; green light had practically no effect.

By varying the length of periods of light, Burger (1939, 1940, 1947, 1953) was able to activate the gonads almost at will. Depending on the length of day involved, the starlings he studied went through successive periods of gonadal activation and retrogression with subsequent renewed activation. By manipulating the periods of light, Emlen (1969) brought about physiological readiness for the spring and fall migrations in the blue bunting. In late spring, using a replica of the springtime night sky, he tested the orientative tendency of two groups of birds. Although an identical replica was used for both groups, the birds prepared for spring migration oriented themselves northwards, those prepared for autumn migration became oriented southwards.

At the ornithological station on the island of Hiddensee, Schildmacher (1938, 1952, 1956) observed that the effective factor causing rutting in birds and mammals is the seasonal variation in the length of daylight. The gonads mature in the course of changes in intensity of light exposure, the male gonad reacting more quickly than the female. If the eyes are shielded from the effect of light, then such maturation does not take place, just as in the case of hypophysectomy.

Detailed studies by Benoit (1934, 1938, 1961a,b, 1964) as well as by Benoit, Walter, and Assenmacher (1950) and Benoit and Assenmacher (1955) demonstrated the effect of ocular light perception on the function of testicles and ovaries. Light had a marked influence on sexual maturation in young male Peking ducks. Sexual maturation occurred first in the group of birds raised under conditions of normal light. Constant darkness had a greater inhibitory effect than artificial constant light (Benoit et al 1959). This reaction, known as the photosexual reflex, revealed that although light is not absolutely necessary for gonadal development, it does stimulate and synchronize gonadal activity (Benoit 1961a). As early as 1938, Benoit postulated the existence of extraretinal receptors for light. In 1964 he attempted to prove their existence in series of experiments that involved covering the eye and cranial regions, enucleation, severing the optic pathway, and cranial trephination. According to his investigations, direct exposure of the retina to light is clearly most effective. By irradiating various portions of the optic system—including the hypothalamus via the orbit after enucleation—increased neurosecretion of the hypothalamus can be achieved, which in turn stimulates gonad growth via the pituitary. Wavelengths of visible red produced the greatest stimulatory effect (Benoit et al 1966).

Since blind Japanese quail respond with evidently normal gonadal function to the stimulus of long periods of light via the skull in spite of the absence of ocular light perception, Homma et al (1972) infer that encephalic photoreception suffices to activate gonadal function. Similar observations were made by Sayler and Wolfson (1968a,b) regarding the Japanese quail and by Menaker and Keatts (1968) regarding the house sparrow. They too consider extraretinal photoreceptors to be sufficient to activate the sexual function in these birds.

Radnot (1954, 1961) also experimented with ducks. By means of periodic nocturnal illumination of the eyes during the gonadal dormancy period, she induced testicular growth and spermogenesis in the drake and ovarian and tubal function as well as egg laying in the duck. Secondary sexual manifestations (e.g., the cockscomb) also developed noticeably in the case of chickens.

Hollwich and Tilgner (1961a,b, 1962, 1963a) continued Benoit's experiments involving the activation of the photosexual reflex in Peking ducks, supplementing them by experiments with monochromatic light of equal intensity (Fig. 48). They reached the following conclusions: irradiation of the ocular region with long-wave monochromatic light strongly stimulates testicular development (red = 16-fold; orange = 6-fold) in contrast to light of short-wave lengths. Paralleling this, histological examination of the testicles reveals stimulation of spermatogenesis.

Studies of the dependence of the sexual function on light in the domestic chicken have had concrete economic implications. Warren and Scott (1936) demonstrated that egg laying is not dependent on the time of day. Additional artificial illumination during the winter months induces maximum laying (Fraps 1959). Regulation of the periods of light can to a large extent control the onset and amount of laying as well as the time of molting (Jöchle 1962). Therefore, in order to obtain the best possible steady production, the poultry farmer keeps his laying hens indoors, exposing them to spring-like light with a high red content (Mehner et al 1962, 1973). With the right combination of illumi-

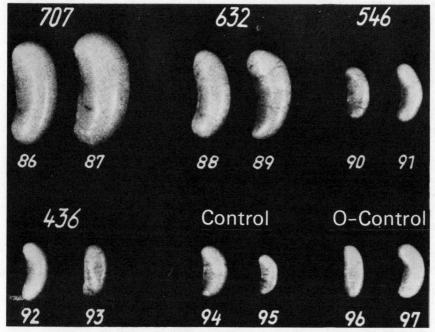

Fig. 48. Testes of five-month-old ducks whose eyes were illuminated for 29 days (total of 12 hours) with monochromatic light of uniform intensity (2.45×10^{-4} W/cm²) but of different wavelength. The numbers above the testes indicate the wavelength, and those below the testes the identity number of the animals.

nation and temperature control, not only does laying activity begin earlier but production is considerably higher too. As opposed to hens raised under normal conditions, 50 to 80 more eggs per hen per laying period can be produced (Kalich 1962).

There were also early attempts to prove that light influences the sexual cycle in mammals. These efforts were hampered by the fact that the experimental animals live under greatly varying conditions of light. Thus, a majority of laboratory animals belongs to the group that becomes active in dusk or darkness—in other words, at a time when thyroid function and metabolism are increasing (Radnot 1961). This in turn influences the activity of the gonads and other endocrine glands. It must also be taken into consideration that some domesticated species such as rats and hamsters, who are seasonal breeders in their natural state, are turned into year-long breeders when subjected to laboratory conditions with controlled environmental factors such as light, climate and diet

(Reiter 1969). These observations are already an indication that in some species certain external factors experienced by the animals in their natural surroundings influence the reproductive cycle. The majority of wild animals reproduces at a specific time of year that is characteristic for the species. In the opinion of many authors, mating time is temporally fixed in the species so that the young are born at that season most favorable for their survival. With domestication, the natural rhythm no longer applies because the environmental conditions have been stabilized; however, fluctuations in light and temperature can produce artificially such periods of reproductive activity or its absence as can be observed in the animals' natural state.

Luce-Clausen et al (1939) discovered that light plays a role in rats' reproductive processes insofar as darkness delays sexual maturation. Fiske (1941) found a retardation of sexual development in rats kept in constant darkness. Constant light increased the content and secretion of the follicle-stimulating hormone* (FSH), but lowered the levels for the luteinizing hormone† (LH). Constant darkness, on the other hand, lowered the FSH content and raised the LH content. Pituitary extract from animals kept in light promoted ovary development to the point of follicle formation as a result of the effect of FSH whereas pituitary extract from animals kept in darkness caused the luteinization of the ovary as a result of the effect of LH. Pomerat (1942) discovered in his series of experiments that extended periods of darkness cause a reduction in the size of rats' ovaries; histologically speaking, however, increased pituitary activity ensues. Pomerat believes this is the mechanism which can produce estrus in nocturnal animals or in animals who rut very early in the year in spite of the absence of light.

Jöchle (1963) discovered a loss of the functional rhythms specific to the two sexes after extended exposure to light. Female rats displayed permanent estrus and hypertrophy of the genital tract as a result of the permanent production of estrogen from cystic follicles; their reproductive capacity, however, was unimpaired. Critchlow's findings (1963) were contradictory. On the one hand, estrus in female rats which followed extended exposure to light did not occur after enucleation; on the other hand, this effect did occur after all connections between the retina and the brain had been destroyed. Critchlow concluded that the eyes are essential for light-induced changes in the pituitary-ovarian system in female rats but that the classical and accessory neural connections behind the optic chiasm are not.

In 1967 Hoffmann also examined the question of the effect of light on the regulation of the estrus cycle in female rats, finding that light appears to be necessary for normal functioning of the pituitary-ovarian system. The findings presented were that blind rats,

i.e., those whose eyes had been surgically removed, did not react to light. Constant light did not cause persistence of their vaginal epithelial cycle nor did inverted diurnal exposure to light alter the onset of epithelial hornification in the vagina. If 21-day-old rats were blinded, or, retaining their eyesight, were placed in absolute darkness, they showed no alterations whatsoever in their cycle up to the age of eight months. However, if animals whose vaginal cycle had already begun had their eyes removed or were placed in absolute darkness, then their cycles became longer after two to three months of darkness; in approximately one-quarter of the animals, the cycle even stopped completely.

Fendler (1967) compared sexual development in newborn rats under conditions of constant illumination and constant darkness. The animals exposed to light showed an increase in the oxytocin content of the neuropituitary and of the hypothalamus as well as hypertrophy of the adrenal glands and testicles.

Further reports on the role of light in activating the gonads in rats were presented by Baker and Ransom (1932), Whitaker (1940), and Lyman (1943). Wurtman and Weisel (1969) studied newborn rats exposed to fluorescent lighting of varying spectral composition. They found that both male and female rats kept under normal white fluorescent lighting for 50 days displayed smaller gonads and a smaller spleen weight than those rats irradiated with artificial light similar to the sun's spectrum (Vita-lite bulbs).

Using lighting filaments for the direct constant exposure of the hypothalamic region to light, Lisk and Kannwischer (1964) produced permanent estrus as well as an increase in the weight of the pituitary and the ovaries in enucleated rats. Clarke and Kennedy (1967) found that temperature and the duration of exposure to light influence the rutting season in voles also. They attributed underdevelopment of the gonads in their experimental animals to involution after estrus or to inhibited development in young animals due to short days. Long days promote

---

*This hormone stimulates the follicles in the female and spermatogenesis in the male.

†This hormone stimulates ovulation in the female and the interstitial cells of Leydig (testosterone) in the male.

weight gain in young animals as well as development of the testicles and accessory sex glands. Summer temperatures heightened this reaction; in mature animals gonad involution did not occur under summer conditions. In this respect, laboratory animals showed a substantially better response than captured voles. Direct measurement of the sex hormones in rats kept in constant darkness revealed that the plasma testosterone level is sharply reduced as compared to the animals kept in light (Kinson and Peat 1971).

Constant light can elicit permanent estrus in older rats more easily than in younger ones. Along with a loss of weight of the ovaries and a weight gain of the uterus, constant light caused an inversion of the FSH and LH serum levels in contrast to control animals (Daane and Parlow 1971). Wurtman and Weisel (1969) found that the spectral composition of the light source used had an effect on rats too. Animals of both sexes developed smaller gonads under cold white fluorescent lighting than under light sources similar to sunlight.

The mouse reacts almost identically to the rat in light experiments. Braden (1957) found accelerated ovulation in light-darkness cycles with a severely shortened phase of darkness. Mice also respond to constant light with permanent estrus (Jöchle 1963). Echave Llanos et al (1967) studied light's influence on the sinusoid rhythm of the mitosis rate in the epithelium of the mammary glands in mice. Light inversion was followed by a phasic shift and increased amplitude in the mitosis rate. Ellendorf and Smidt (1971) exposed newborn mice to varying light conditions. They found that constant darkness as opposed to constant light and to light-darkness alternation inhibit body growth and sexual development.

Bloch (1964, 1965) reported on his studies of genital function in mice. Frequent manifestations of disintegration of the ova and follicles and a continuous descent of the testes were observed under conditions of constant light and constant darkness as well as of irradiation with 10 hours of artificial light (300 lux) alternating with a 14-hour confinement to darkness. The alterations in reaction observed in constant light and constant darkness and the increase in the weight of the pituitary did not appear, however, with intermittent exposure to light.

Light caused a weight gain in the testicles of male golden hamsters (Radnot 1961). Gaston and Menaker (1967) were able to demonstrate a positive correlation between periods of light and size of the gonads in the case of adult animals only; he found no correlation between body weight and testicle weight. Reiter (1969) reported gonadal involution in male and female golden hamsters within a few weeks following enucleation. Gonadal involution occurs under conditions of constant darkness: spermatogenesis stops, tubular epithelial cells and accessory sex glands degenerate, and testosterone production is reduced (Desjardins et al 1971). Frehn and Liu (1970) studied the influence of temperature and varying periods of light on the golden hamster's testicular development. Fourteen hours of daylight and an unchanging summer temperature did not cause any alteration in testicular weight; however, reducing the period of light to eight hours led to a testicular weight loss of 90 percent.

Exposure to cold also caused a rapid weight loss. After reaching a low point in the eighth week of the experiment, weight returned to its original level in the 16th week when the longer period of light treatment was used. Frehn and Liu see the results of this experiment as proof that cold as well as the shortening of periods of light influences the nature of testicular function. Elliott et al (1972) exposed golden hamsters to a short-day rhythm with unvarying six-hour periods of light but with lengthening periods of darkness reaching a final total of 60 hours. The animals' diurnal activity was checked by measuring their use of a treadwheel. In cycles lasting one or two entire days, the short day led to testicular regression whereas in cycles lasting one and a half or two and a half days testicle weight was maintained. These results indicate that light exerts an influence on the gonads via an internal circadian clock.

In 1940 Marshal investigated the effect of varying intensities of irradiation on the occurrence and duration of estrus, finding that light's ability to cause the premature onset of the cycle correlates with the intensity of irradiation. Light also had the effect of causing the testes of the male ferret to descend as early as December.

In rabbits, cats, and ferrets, ovulation occurs in response to the secretion of gonadotropin after mating. This mechanism can be used to test gonadotropin-inhibiting substances. Farrell et al (1968) found that the ovulation induced by mating did not occur in the light-deficient seasons in particular but practically always took place in spring. Using this knowledge they caused a practically constant readiness for ovulation by means of supplemental artificial lighting approximating the light of springtime. Smelser et al (1934) studied the effect of additional light on the rate of ovulation after mating had taken place. A comparison between rabbits kept in light and those kept in darkness revealed no additional stimulatory effect of light on ovulation. On the other hand, if young rabbits are kept in constant darkness, a significant retardation of testicle development may be observed after two months; however, no difference in body growth can be observed (Radnot and Strobl 1964). Faure et al (1971) exposed female rabbits of varying stages of sexual maturity to irradiation with fluorescent lighting. In the spring and fall they discovered that after at least ten days of exposure to light for 14 hours a day there was marked follicular maturation which in winter could be obtained only by exposure to longer periods of light. But young rabbits approaching sexual maturity displayed, especially in winter, a more rapid reaction up to the time of ovulation. Walter and his co-workers (1968) reported on photoperiodic regulation of sexual activity in male and female rabbits. Fifteen males and 30 females were divided into three groups and were exposed to light for 8, 12, and 16 hours each within a 24-hour period for the 9 months that the experiment lasted. The mean weight of the testicles was highest for the males exposed to the shortest periods of light (8 hours) and lowest for those with the longest periods of light (16 hours). The same pattern was true for body weight. The spermatozoid count of the epididymis was higher in the rabbits with an 8-hour than with a 16-hour period of light. The results were exactly the reverse for the females: 44 percent of the females with a 16-hour period of light accepted the male during the experiment whereas 22 percent with an 8-hour period of light always rejected the male.

Estrus normally appears in the spring in female ferrets, but when they are kept under continuous illumination estrus can appear at any time of year. On the other hand, estrus appears at the normal time in the following spring in ferrets blinded in summer and fall, regardless of prevailing light conditions. Estrus did not occur in mature ferrets kept under short-day conditions during the summer. When the same animal was then transferred to long-day conditions, estrus did occur. The appearance of the first estrus in young ferrets is normally limited to spring. Ferrets born and raised under continuous illumination have their first estrus at any time of year. Shortened periods of daylight accelerate the first appearance of estrus; artificially long days delay it. When immature ferrets were transferred from a short to a long day, the first estrus was sharply accelerated or indefinitely delayed, depending on the age of the ferret experiencing the change in light conditions. These observations do not indicate the existence of an endogenic rhythm period which determines the time at which estrus will occur, but they do denote that environmental light is the main regulatory factor. Age and estrus history also influence the ferret's response to changes in environmental light conditions (Thorpe 1967).

Hammond (1973) studied a large colony of ferrets for twelve years, observing a total of 1,000 animals under the influence of changing conditions of temperature and light. He modified the general assumption that long periods of light stimulate gonadal maturation and activity by his discovery that ferrets must be full grown before light can exert its regulatory influence. It is natural to infer from this that photoregulation inhibits the ability to reproduce mainly at those seasons when it would be inappropriate. Similar examples are offered by the hare and deer, who conceive in autumn but do not give birth until a favorable season. Ferrets raised in artificial and constant light from birth on reach sexual maturity several months later than normal; under long-day conditions, they never reach it. However, if the animals have already attained sexual maturity, full gonadal activity can be sustained for almost the entire year by an unvarying light rhythm.

A secondary sexual characteristic in deer and red deer, the antlers, shows an annual increase based on a firm formula. Von Schumacher-Marienfrid (1939) was struck by the fact that the number of prize-winning deer antlers awarded at the Tirolian Hunt Show varied from year to year. Antler growth in the roebuck takes place during the light-deficient months of November to March. Von Schumacher-Marienfrid studied the relevant factors of snow cover, temperature, and duration of sunshine, reaching the conclusion that the number of hours of sunlight is the most important factor in new growth

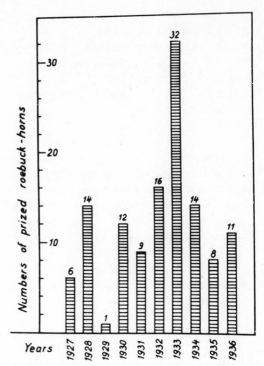

Fig. 50. Numbers of prized horns of the roebucks for the years 1927 through 1936, at the hunting show of Tyrol (Schumacher von Marienfrid).

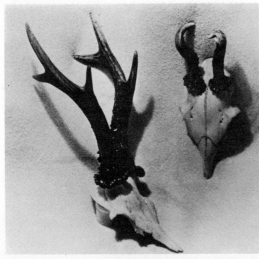

Fig. 49. Left: Normal developed horns. Right: Deformed horns in consequence of insufficient sunshine during the winter months.

of the antlers. Thus, a sunny winter was followed by a greater number of prize-winning antlers. The red deer is not subject to these fluctuations, since his antlers develop from April to June, at a time of year when the hours of sunlight are considerably higher than in winter even if weather conditions are unfavorable (Figs. 49, 50).

Domesticated mammals are subject to a yearly reproductive cycle (Ortavant 1973). The ram displays maximal testicle weight and the most intensive spermatogenesis from summer to late fall. The rate of ovulation in the ewe declines to a minimum during the winter months, rising to a maximum from summer to late fall. In experiments with light, the ram showed the greatest sexual activity as the length of the days decreased; the ewe's gonadal activity was reduced by half in keeping with the year's photorhythm. The duration of periods of fertility is clearly dependent on the degree of latitude; the farther north the species is domiciled, the shorter the duration of estrus. Higher temperatures lead to hypoxia of the germinative tissue. The thermosensitive germ cells are inhibited. Ortavant generalized that long periods of light and higher environmental temperatures have a negative influence on fertility in domesticated mammals, whereas days lasting ten to 12 hours and moderate temperatures bring the greatest success in livestock breeding.

Effects on Humans

It is difficult to use human subjects in direct experiments involving the influence of light on the gonads. It is virtually impractical to expose subjects to experimental light conditions for a sufficiently long period. There is, however, the alternative possibility of "natural" experiments with light such as are provided by blindness, polar night, and change in light intensity depending on the degree of latitude.

Jafarey et al (1970) tried to explain the relatively early occurrence of menarche in countries with a warmer climate (e.g., India) as opposed to countries with a colder climate (e.g., the United States) by pointing out the greater use of artificial lighting in the colder zone. This lengthening of the periods of light might have a retarding effect. Radnot (1961) reported the suspension of ovulation during the polar night; Marx (1946) noted a decline in libido and potency in the polar winter. Studies by Benoit (1961a,b) showed a 30 percent increase of ejaculated sperm in American students from August to March and a large increase in women's estrogen excretion in the urine from January to March. Parkes (1968), in less detailed investigations on the other hand, did not find amenorrhea in Eskimo women during the polar winter; there was even a slight increase in the number of conceptions.

Most authors agree that sexual development begins earlier in blind girls than in their normal-sighted peers. Zacharias and Wurtman (1964, 1969b) examined girls born prematurely who had developed retrolental fibroplasia due to hyperoxygenation and to being underweight during the newborn period and thus were virtually blind. In comparison to normal-sighted people born prematurely, the less residual vision remained the earlier menarche occurred in this group. Full-term babies who became blind during the first year of life were also included in the study, since the influence of premature birth or of retrolental fibroplasia on sexual development could not be totally excluded. Girls were selected for the experimental group if blindness was confined merely to the eyeball, not including neuroendocrine structures, and if any other pathological process influencing sexual development could be eliminated. Excluding all factors with the exception of the absence of photostimulus, the authors noted a marked premature menarche in the full-term blind girls too. Magee et al (1970) reached similar findings for girls blind at birth. Menarche occurred earlier both in those subjects who were totally blind and in those who retained a slight degree of light perception than in those who could still perceive shadows. These data show very clearly that physiologically normal sexual development in humans is a process functionally dependent on light perception via the eye just as it is in other mammals.

Kaloud (1970) observed the relatively early maturity in blind girls as well as the fact that they generally are retarded in body growth although menarche and the secondary sex characteristics appear fully in keeping with their age.

Various authors have tried to clarify the question of light's regulatory effect on the menstrual cycle. Kienast (1955) found irregularities in the cycles of blind women which were all the more pronounced if blindness occurred during adolescence. Fertility and libido seemed not to be affected, however. Kienast regarded menstrual irregularities as a manifestation of autonomic dysregulation due to changes in psychic state rather than as the result of the absence of photoperception. Strobel and Dorschner (1956) questioned 60 blind women—some with residual vision, some with amaurosis—about anomalies in their menstrual cycle. They did not find any connection between photoperception and menstrual cycle, since in the case of only six women was blindness the sole cause of irregularity. Recent more detailed studies by von Schumann (1973) seem to verify light's effect on the female sexual cycle. Less than ten percent out of 30 women who became blind early in life had regular menstruation; the rate for women with cycle fluctuations of more than 60 days was nine times higher than for normal-sighted control persons. Becoming blind during the age of sexual maturity led to irregularities and amenorrheal periods lasting for months, although periods had previously been regular. Hypermenorrhea and leukorrhea almost always occurred.

Knaus (1950) found that there is an increase in psychoses related to the menstrual cycle during light-deficient months as a result of an inadequate supply of light to the pituitary; he also found that European women often experience temporary sterility in the tropics as a result of the overly intense effect of light. These observations point to a functional relationship between the eye and pituitary.

Over a period of five years, Timonen and co-workers (1964) in Helsinki studied the rate of conception in a considerable number of women whose vaginal smears and biopsies indicated cysts and other forms of cell proliferation. They compared their statistical findings with the monthly measurements of sunlight taken by the Central Meteorological Bureau, discovering that the number of conceptions increased with increasing sunlight and tumorlike cell proliferation, designated as hyperplasia, decreased. The results were reversed during the dark months.

Reinberg (1974) examined a young woman who had spent almost three months in a cave with only the dim light of a miner's lamp. She measured her temperature daily for one year before and one year after this experience. Previously she had lived a 24-hour day and had a menstrual cycle of 29 days. With the absence of daylight during her stay in the cave, her day was lengthened to 24.6 hours and her menstrual cycle shortened to 25.7 days. After the end of her confinement to darkness, it took approximately one year until her cycle returned to 29 days.

Kaiser and Halberg (1962) reported that in 60 percent of women, labor begins in the night, reaching a high point around 3 A.M. Most stillbirths or cases in which infants died shortly after birth occurred in the late afternoon. These findings imply that the circadian phase plays an extremely important role in a healthy pregnancy.

Perhaps the effects of light on the neuroendocrine system can also explain some of the stereotyped views concerning temperament and climate, e.g., the melancholy Danes or the high-spirited Italians. Perhaps it is not only the cold but also the deficiency of sunlight that depresses the spirits of people in high latitudes.

The beginning of labor also seems to be subject to the influence of light. Thus, Hosemann (1946) found that in 10,000 births labor began around midnight in a majority of cases. Schlegel and co-workers (1966) observed 1,800 healthy women between the ages of 18 and 30 who had experienced a normal pregnancy. Delivery proceeded without medication or surgery. The researchers found that labor showed a marked and quite regular diurnal fluctuation, with a maximum of cases occurring at 2 A.M. and a minimum at noon. Women giving birth for the first time displayed this rhythm more clearly than those who had given birth before.

Not only constant illumination or constant darkness affects sexual processes; so does a single photoimpulse. Engelmann (1969) found a circadian rhythm in the emergence of drosophilia from the pupa state. A single photoimpulse, depending on the circadian time at which it is given, causes a phasic shift in the hatching maxima. The maximal effect of the photoimpulse is described by the following equation: $E = 10^4$ erg/cm^2.

All these factors caused Hollwich and Dieckhues (1968, 1971d, 1974b) to investigate the sex hormones of the anterior lobe of the pituitary. Gonadotropic excretion in the urine can be regarded as one of the parameters for gonadotropic activity of the pituitary's anterior lobe. Studies of this were made on the one hand in the blind as compared with the normal-sighted and on the other hand in patients who had been practically blind for months as a result of cataracts in both eyes and who then had regained their sight after successful surgery. By examining the same patient under unchanging conditions of environment and diet, the content of the luteinizing hormone in the serum or urine could be measured, first presurgically in the practically blind state and then postsurgically with restored sight. The authors demonstrated that in the case of intact ocular photoperception, light stimulates gonadotropin incretion in humans via the "energetic portion of the visual pathway" (Hollwich 1948).

The stimulatory effect of light on testosterone could also be demonstrated. When light's entry into the eye was blocked (in the case of the blind), testosterone excretion in the urine was significantly lower than in the normal-sighted (Lenau et al 1976).

In anamnestic inquiries, von Schumann learned that the sexual potency of blind men declined upon the loss of sight but that libido remained the same or even increased.

Since light and especially the light–darkness alternation have been proven to have an extremely strong effect on sexual functioning, there was great interest in locating an endogenic rhythm of the sexual hormones caused by the day–night alternation.

After the introduction of radioimmunological methods for identifying the gonadotropins, which are very fragile and therefore difficult to measure, Faiman and Ryan (1967) were able to establish a diurnal rhythm for FSH, with a peak at 5 A.M. and a minimum in the early afternoon. Leyendecker and Saxena (1970) published slightly differing results; they found that LH also displayed pronounced diurnal fluctuations. Further studies by Alford et al (1973) and Osterman et al (1974) confirmed the incretion rhythm for gonadotropins in both men and women. In testing a diurnally rhythmic reaction of gonadotropin secretion to the LH-releasing factor, Schwarzstein et al (1975) discovered varying values, but they were unable to establish a rhythm in the basic secretion. Kapen et al (1974) used the nocturnal rise in the concentration of LH serum during puberty as an experimental model to test the influence of a sleep-waking inversion on LH secretion. When measurements were made at 20-minute intervals, they found that the increase in LH secretion also occurred in sleep during the day, whereas during nocturnal wakefulness a heightened LH level was maintained. A single occurrence of sleep (and thus light) inversion was not capable of suppressing this endocrine rhythm. A circadian period was likewise reported for testosterone, with a matutinal maximum around 6 A.M. and a nocturnal minimum around 10 P.M. (De Lacerda et al 1973; Lincoln et al 1974; Nieschlag 1974; Smals et al 1974). Judd et al (1974) proved that the nocturnal increase in testosterone has its sole source in the testicles and follows LH incretion. Alford et al (1973) reported a circadian rhythm for estradiol.

11
Light and Adrenal and Pituitary Functions

The adrenal gland is an organ central to the regulation of metabolism. It consists of two parts of varying embryonal origin: the adrenal medulla stemming from the ectoderm and the adrenal cortex stemming from the mesoderm. Although the functioning of the medullar portion can be assumed by the sympathetic ganglia present in the rest of the organism, life without the adrenal cortex is impossible, as shall be seen presently.

Thus far, over 50 different hormonal compounds from the adrenal cortex have been isolated. Cortisol and corticosterone are the most important ones among the glucocorticoids and aldosterone among the mineralocorticoids. In addition, there is a significant amount of secretion of androgens.

Cortisol's primary effect is its role in carbohydrate, protein, and fat metabolism. Its ergotropic function is seen in a shift in the metabolic condition from the constructive phase to an increasingly functional one. In gluconeogenesis a redistribution of glycogen from the periphery to the liver takes place along with a neogenesis of sugar from protein, which results in a reduction of the body's protein content. The protein cata-

bolic effect is accompanied by a rise in protein metabolites. Cortisol has only a slight influence on electrolyte and water metabolism as well as on fat metabolism. On the other hand, it has a lasting influence on the hematopoietic system, leading to leukocytosis with eosinopenia and lymphopenia, to an increase in thrombocytes and erythrocytes, and to a reduction in lymphatic tissue. Its inhibitory influence on the proliferation of connective tissue and of all reactions of the mesenchymal system has broad therapeutic applications. Corticosterone has far-reaching biological effects similar to cortisol, but it displays mineralocorticoid qualities.

Cortisol and ACTH

For a long time the influence of the hormones of the adrenal cortex on the organism could be traced only indirectly through their presence in the lymphocytes and eosinophils circulating in the blood and in the steroid hormonal metabolites in the urine. Pincus (1943) was the first to describe a diurnal rhythm in the excretion of 17-ketosteroids*; he took this phenomenon as the sign of a cyclic adrenal function. Refined methods of hormonal measurement of blood plasma enabled Bliss et al (1953) to measure the level of plasma 17-hydroxycorticosterone (17-OHCS) at different times of day. They came to the conclusion that the hormone level reaches its high point in the early morning, to decline in the course of the day and the night. Detailed studies made by other authors at more frequent intervals showed that in addition to a matutinal peak around 8 A.M. there was another rise in the plasma level in the course of the afternoon, although a considerably smaller one (Perkoff et al 1959; Orth et al 1967; Orth and Island 1969; Migeon et al 1956; Retienne et al 1965).

Migeon et al (1956) observed that 17-OHCS excretion in the urine follows the same course as the plasma concentration, but approximately two hours later. Various authors describe a diurnal pattern of corticoid excretion in the urine. Common to the 24-hour rhythm is a maximum between 2 and 4 A.M. and a minimum at noon (Bartter et al 1962; Wisser et al 1973; Giedke and Fatranska 1974; Köbberling and von Zurmühlen 1974). Under conditions of both constant light and constant darkness, the circadian rhythm of excretion in the urine was maintained; in constant darkness total excretion was greater, the maximum occurring slightly later (Fatranska 1971). The close connection between the level of plasma cortisol and sleep could not be established in the case of night workers who slept during the day (Migeon et al 1956). For them as well as for daytime workers, the pattern of hormonal secretion remained an independent endocrine rhythm, even after a lengthy period of habituation to their work schedule. A connection with the day-night alternation had to be assumed, however, after Flink and Doe (1959) had studied the behavior of steroid excretion following an airplane flight involving a time change of nine hours. They discovered that the original rhythm re-

mained the same initially but then in the course of nine days adapted itself completely to the new time conditions.

Sharp et al (1961) traced alterations in the endogenic rhythm under conditions of a polar summer in a person whose sleep-activity pattern was reversed from time to time. In the constant light of the polar summer the adaptation as well as readaptation of the rhythm of the hormones of the adrenal cortex took place within a week. These authors conclude from this that the factors determining the rhythm are environment and adaptation.

Orth among others (1967, 1969) further investigated the influence of these factors. Healthy subjects submitted themselves to an artificial period of light and darkness which involved their sleeping while it was light and being awake during a dark period which lasted as long as their normal sleeping time; their hormonal level was measured hourly under these conditions. At the end of the period of darkness, all subjects reacted with a marked peak in 17-OHCS secretion. If the nocturnal dark phase was extended beyond the time of awakening, then the matutinal peak did not occur until it became light, not at the usual time of awakening in darkness. If the subjects received only one afternoon hour of illumination, then the matutinal peak was delayed and was smaller, to be followed by an exaggerated peak when exposure to light commenced. Even after a period of light lasting for three weeks, there was a constant matutinal rise in the level of corticosteroid. Orth and Island (1969) found indications in three blind persons of an autonomous corticosteroid rhythm which is not dependent on the sleep-waking period and can, in addition, shift.

Hellmann et al (1970) used two healthy men for experiments with very short time intervals. In order to eliminate disturbing influences associated with the experiment as much as possible, the subjects were prepared for weeks in advance for a constant sleep-waking rhythm and the manipulations associated with the sleep laboratory. With the aid of radioactively marked cortisol, cor-

*Excretory product of androgen (testosterone).

tisol secretion was measured at quarter-hour intervals at the same time as the sleeping state was electroencephalographically recorded. In this manner, the already familiar peak in the late, matutinal phase of sleep could be divided into several secretory peaks closely connected to phases of light sleep. Further studies of the diurnal secretory pattern revealed that there are several individual peaks occurring at different times, always followed by a lowering in the level of plasma cortisol. On the basis of these results, Hellmann and his co-workers questioned the theory of steady state secretion advocated by many writers; however, their very findings indicate that the degree of central nervous system (CNS) stimulation (stress, sleep, light, and so on) directly influences cortisol secretion. These authors are also supported by studies of ACTH secretion.

The influence of external factors on the creation of a corticosteroid rhythm was shown in the findings mentioned above made under conditions of a polar summer. This can also be demonstrated in the growing child from the time of birth on. As the child matures, an increasing amount of his sleep will occur at night. Paralleling this, the daily fall in plasma corticosteroid is established in the infant, starting at zero in the full-term newborn and reaching the adult rhythm in the older infant (Franks 1967). The development in the infant of a mature sleep-waking cycle such as is found in the adult precedes the maturation of the corticosteroid rhythm by several months.

Aschoff et al (1971) found this rhythm to be extremely stable since experiments conducted in caves, where light was absent, did not cause any alteration or time shift. Vernikos-Danellis et al (1972) followed the development of the diurnal cortisol rhythm during almost two months of bed rest under invariable light conditions. The amplitude of the cortisol peak was reduced, it is true, but the rhythm was sustained without interruption. In contrast, easy bed exercises serving as a synchronizing training effect made no difference. A strict diet for two or three weeks

also had no effect on the cortisol rhythm (Reinberg et al 1974); neither did the unvarying oral administration of glucose or a mixture of egg, milk, and sugar (Krieger et al 1971). Age, sex, and hospitalization had no effect on the corticosteroid rhythm.

Experiments have been performed concerning the corticosteroid rhythm in nocturnal laboratory rats. Fiske and Leeman (1964) studied the effect of light on adrenal function and found that female rats, in contrast to males, lost weight after exposure to constant light. The corticoid rhythm typical for rats, with its low matutinal and high evening plasma corticoid level, almost disappeared with constant light. A noteworthy discovery by these authors is the appearance of neurosecretory activity in the nucleus supraopticus and paraventricularis coinciding with the beginning of diurnal corticoid rhythm in the third week of a rat's life. Scheving and Pauly (1966) exposed rats to varying light conditions, observing a 24-hour rhythm of the plasma corticoid level when there was a light-darkness alternation; in this case corticoid concentration correlated directly with the duration of light periods. Constant light and constant darkness caused an autonomic rhythm to come about. A lengthened light-darkness rhythm representing an increase in the length of the natural day (where one "day" equaled 36 or 48 hours) did not alter the endocrine rhythm in rats. Their physical activity (running) and plasma corticosterone exhibited a periodicity of 36 or 48 hours; the experimental animals retained a clear endogenic rhythm, with a slightly lengthened duration of between 23.5 and 26.2 hours.

Upon carefully analyzing the amplitudes of both factors, Szafarczyk et al (1974) find that the endogenic adrenal cortex rhythm proceeds autonomically when there are radical changes in photoindicators of time and, in addition, shows greater stability than the activity rhythm.

Hollwich and Dieckhues (1971d) observed the behavior of the 17-ketosteroid level in the urine of rabbits exposed to a 38-day period of darkness (Fig. 51). The steroid rhythm, similar to that in humans, became abnormal in amplitude and duration, returning however to its normal physiological course after three days of day-night alternation.

Kolpakov et al (1974) described the annual pattern of corticoid and aldosterone secretion, using the hibernating Siberian ground squirrel for their tests. The activity cycle of the ground squirrel is characterized by a very short period of intense activity and a long period of hibernation. At the beginning of the active period in May are found the highest values for the production of both hormones in terms of nuclear size and rate of absorption of radioactively marked metabolites in the zona fasciculata and glomerulosa of the adrenal cortex. In June and July there is a regression of the adrenal cortex, with a reduction in corticoid production and size of the cell nuclei. They also found a decreasing sensitivity of the adrenal cortex when stimulated by ACTH: the strongest reaction took place in May; in July it declined by two-thirds. When experiments were made during hibernation, there was a conspicuous increase in activity from month to month as the length of the days increased. Given the seasonally varying sensitivity of the adrenal cortex to ACTH stimulation and its annual pattern of secretion, Kolpakov and his co-workers inferred the adrenal cortex's central role in the regulation of a year-long cycle.

Since the introduction of technical methods for the measurement of ACTH level, numerous studies of ACTH rhythm have been made. Berson and Yalow (1968) observed irregular secretion patterns of ACTH in healthy subjects, finding however the lowest values in the late evening hours. Hellmann et al (1970) measured the plasma corticoid level at quarter-hour intervals, inferring from the elimination pattern of cortisol and their knowledge of the half life of ACTH (Orth et al 1967) that there is a brief peaklike release of the corticotropic hormone. They excluded the possiblity of continuous secretion since episodic peaks of ACTH and corticoid levels were evident. Krieger et al (1967) assume that the sharp matutinal rise of plasma corticosteroids and ACTH repre-

sents a daily, neurally caused release, which occurs only during a critical time of day, of corticotropin and the releasing factor and consequently of ACTH. The subsequent secretion of ACTH and the corticosteroids is seen as a response to the metabolic state and other external or internal influences upon CRF release. A three-hour sleep-waking rhythm did not interfere with the endogenic 24-hour rhythm of cortisol secretion. Even after ten days the circadian cortisol rhythm, earlier recognized as regulatory, was clearly maintained, but a three-hour period was superimposed upon it (Weitzman et al 1974).

The mineralocorticoid aldosterone, whose connection with the renal tubules will be discussed later in more detail, appears to be another important steroid hormone released by the adrenal cortex in a circadian rhythm. Williams et al (1972) described a diurnal rhythm independent of body position and dietary factors, but the time intervals they used were too long for them to prove the existence of a definite circadian rhythm. Katz et al (1972) tested two resting experimental subjects every 20 minutes and found a secretion rhythm similar to that for cortisol. The number of subjects was too small, however, to provide conclusive evidence.

Vagnucci et al (1974) published a similar study of four subjects who continued normal physical activity and followed a low-salt diet. The authors report a rise in aldosterone production with the onset of sleep; during the waking hours the frequency, duration, and amplitudes of secretory rhythms varied. There was at the same time a correlation with renin activity but little with the excretion of cortisol and corticosteroids. In later experiments, especially during the second half of sleep and shortly after awakening, Katz et al (1975) found peaks in the excretion of aldosterone and a relatively dormant period during the evening hours paralleling the secretion rhythm of cortisol. In the authors' opinion this shows a pronounced dependence of both hormones, aldosterone and cortisol, on ACTH excretion, although the aldosterone rhythm remained nearly the same after dexamethasone suppression by

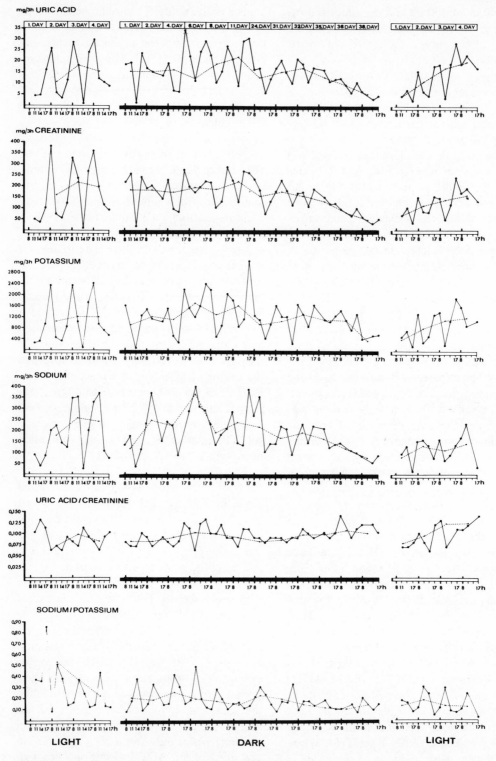

(A)

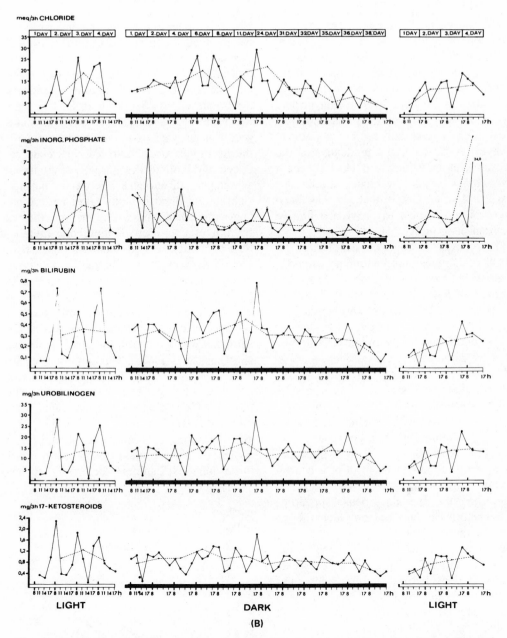

Fig. 51 A and B. Circadian rhythm of metabolites (urine) in light and darkness: Normal circadian rhythm of 15 rabbits during a four-day period of normal day and night conditions. During the next 38-day period with constant darkness the circadian rhythm is disturbed. Amplitude and average excretion of metabolites continue to decrease with the length of period of darkness. Restoration of normal day and night conditions brings about a normalization within three days (Hollwich and Dieckhues 1971).

ACTH and cortisol, indicating an external regulation of aldosterone. Kowarski et al (1975) similarly found a slight correlation between aldosterone secretion and cortisol rhythm. Secretory peaks occurred especially after arising but also during normal physical activity. The authors were not able to establish a clear-cut secretory pattern, however. Aside from the tendency for the lowest secretory values to occur between 4 P.M. and 4 A.M. and the highest amplitudes between 4 A.M. and 4 P.M., it has been impossible up to now to prove a definitive circadian periodicity.

The reported findings on ACTH and 17-OHCS in humans, unlike that in animals, seems to indicate a subordinate role for the influence of light. If the temporarily blind, who represent "natural" experimental subjects (in other words, persons whose ocular perception of light has been temporarily hindered by cataracts), are examined, surprising results are revealed. Orth and Island (1969) found indications in two blind persons of an autonomous corticoid rhythm not connected to the sleep-waking rhythm. Krieger et al (1971) found abnormal corticoid secretory patterns in the plasma of 13 blind patients whose blindness was not of a central nervous genesis. Along with the matutinal peak, abnormal secondary peaks appeared; the secretory rhythms did not recur in the same manner every day.

Extensive studies by Hollwich and Dieckhues (1967a, 1971a, 1972a, 1974b) of cataract patients before and after removal of the cataracts showed a significant influence of light perception on cortisol secretion and rhythm. They found that patients blind because of cataracts showed a lowering of the matutinal peak and a lower curve pattern than the normal sighted (Fig. 52). Excretion of cortisol metabolites in the urine was significantly lowered. After surgery, with the return of normal light perception, the amplitudes of the peaks in the serum as well as total excretion rose to the level of the normal sighted. In addition, Hollwich and Dieckhues (1972) found a general reduction and flattening of the curves for the level of

plasma cortisol in the blind in contrast to the pronounced matutinal rise in the normal sighted caused by the entry of light in the morning hours (Fig. 53). Hollwich concluded from this that ocular perception of light stimulates pituitary-adrenal cortex function. This explains the fact that basal secretion as well as excretory maxima for the hormones of the adrenal cortex are reduced in the blind. Furthermore, they found significant differences between normal-sighted and blind patients (after and before cataract operations) as far as the diurnal rhythm of excretion of metabolic metabolites dependent on cortisol was concerned.

In order to find out whether light's stimulatory effect on metabolism takes place in direct relation to ACTH secretion or whether there is a primary insufficiency of adrenal cortex, ACTH's role in lowering eosinophils was studied in the blind (Hollwich and Dieckhues 1967a). The amount of eosinophils was measured at different times of day in 15 blind patients with cataracts. The next day the same tests were repeated, with intramuscular injections of ACTH being given at noon. According to expectation, no eosinopenia was found in the morning hours in any of the 15 subjects before the ACTH

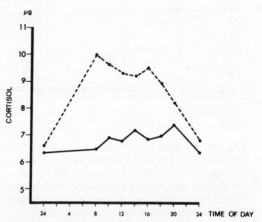

Fig. 52. Compares the difference in the diurnal rhythm cortisol levels in ten cataract patients before and after cataract surgery. After restoration of normal ocular light perception there was a marked increase in the morning plasma content of cortisol. Solid line, before surgery; broken line, after surgery (Hollwich and Dieckhues 1971).

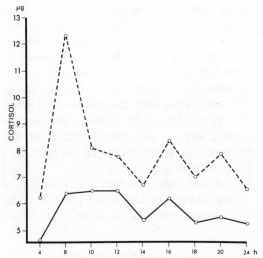

μg

Fig. 53. Average of circadian variation of plasma cortisol levels in 50 blind persons compared with the average of 35 persons with normal ocular light perception. The increase of cortisol in plasma in the morning in the normal patients is less pronounced in the blind. In normal patients the average basic secretion is 9.2 μg/ml, while in blind persons this was reduced to 6.24 μg/ml. Broken line, normal sighted; solid line, blind (Hollwich and Dieckhues).

injection (see Fig. 36). The injection, however, triggered immediately a drop in eosinophils amounting to a mean value of 52 percent of the original value. This positive result of the ACTH test in the blind indicates normal functioning of the adrenal cortex and points to an absence of ACTH secretion in the pituitary as a result of the lack of light stimulation. After surgery and the restoration of light's entry into the eye, physiological matutinal eosinopenia again appeared.

Catecholamines

Little research has been done on the effect of light on the synthesis, release, and metabolism of catecholamines, although it is known that the catecholamines (noradrenalin, dopamin, and adrenalin) fulfill important functions in neural and endocrine terms (Wurtman 1966). The only study in this connection was done by Januszkiewicz and Wo-

cial (1960), who observed a total lack of diurnal fluctuations of noradrenalin in the blind. Hollwich and co-workers (1969), Dieckhues (1974), and Hollwich and Dieckhues (1975) studied the diurnal fluctuations of catecholamines as well as their catabolite vanillin-mandelic acid (VMA)* in the urine of the blind, the normal sighted, the normal sighted after being kept in darkness, and cataract patients before and after surgery. The results showed that there are significant differences in catecholamine metabolism in the normal sighted and in patients unable to perceive light. In a comparison between 60 blind and 25 normal-sighted persons, they found the excretion of adrenalin, noradrenalin, and vanillin-mandelic acid lowered to a highly significant degree in the urine of the blind (Fig. 54). The same was true for cataract patients before (blind) and after (with sight) surgery (Fig. 55).

As research has shown, a short, six-day confinement to darkness in the case of normal-sighted experimental subjects leads to an only slight levelling of fluctuations in VMA. The constant absence of ocular light stimulation (the blind), on the other hand, lowers the amplitudes and leads in part to a complete loss of the diurnal rhythm.

Kriebel (1970) observed an autonomic periodicity of the hormones of the adrenal medulla in a healthy experimental subject. Following the exclusion of all time indicators there developed a constant, autonomous rhythm of about 26 hours which showed a phasic shift in relation to body temperature and the 17-OHCS rhythm. Wisser et al (1973) studied the urinary excretion of catecholamines and their metabolites in six male subjects at intervals of three hours during the course of a day with a fixed schedule. Food and beverages that stimulate catecholamines were avoided. Although varying peaks in amplitude were revealed, the researchers observed a pronounced rhythm, with noon maxima and nocturnal minima for catecholamines and VMA, which ran three

*A catabolite of adrenalin that is secreted in the urine.

hours behind the corticoid rhythm. The comprehensive study by Descovich et al (1973) of 106 test subjects ranging in age from 20 to 99 confirmed the diurnal rhythm established previously. Age does not influence rhythm or phasic state but only amplitude in the form of a reduction in excretion.

Fatranska (1971) published further research in which she included a normal-sighted control group in an experiment with darkness. The blind subjects exhibited a daily pattern of VMA excretion in the urine similar to that found in earlier experiments. Amplitude was significantly lower than for

those with normal sight. Six days of constant darkness also reduced excretory amplitudes in the normal sighted, although they did remain higher than for the blind exposed to light-darkness conditions. Although Neal et al (1968) had already reported a lowering of VMA excretion with minimal physical activity and a reduction in activity in the normal sighted kept in constant darkness, on the basis of measurements of blind persons pursuing normal activity in a home for the blind it may be concluded that the reduction of diurnal fluctuations for VMA was caused by the absence of light. Levine et al (1973)

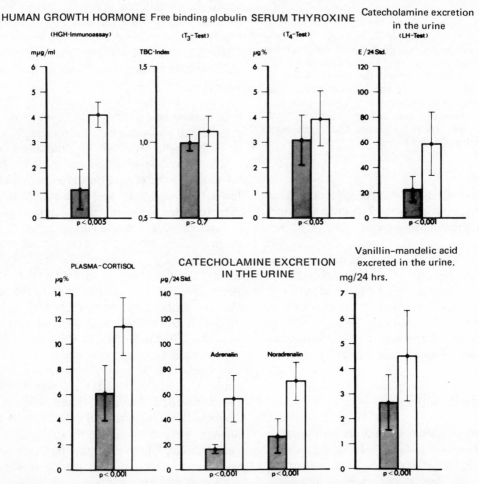

Fig. 54. Various hormone studies were performed on 60 blind persons in comparison with 25 normal-sighted control subjects. With the exception of the thyroxine-binding globulin (T_3 test) lowered values—ranging from significant to highly significant—were found in the blind. Shaded bar, blind (n = 60); open bar, normal sighted (n = 25) (Hollwich and Dieckhues 1975).

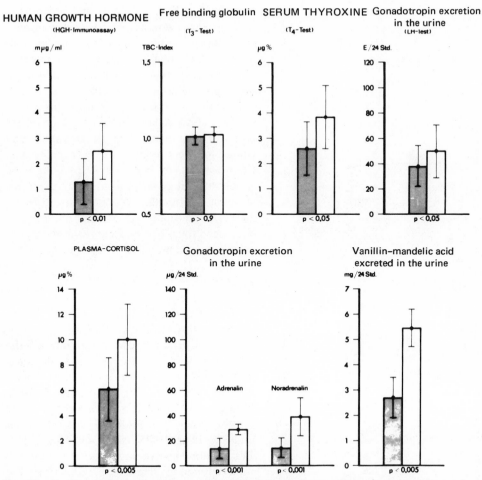

Fig. 55. In 20 cataract patients in a state of blindness before surgery, the values for various hormones were subnormal. After surgery and the sight restoration, these values became normal in the same patients. Except in the case of the thyroxine-binding globulin, significant to highly significant differences were found before and after cataract surgery. Shaded bar, before surgery; open bar, after surgery (Hollwich and Dieckhues 1975).

traced the development of endocrine rhythms in a three-year-old boy who had had to undergo enucleation because of retinoblastoma in both eyes. (It should be noted that one-fourth of the patients with retinoblastoma show elevated VMA excretion levels.) After double enucleation no desynchronization of the circadian systems was observed. The researchers interpret this as the result of adaptation to the protracted lost vision and entry of light. Giedke and Fatranska (1974) studied six male subjects under strict experimental conditions in order to determine the influence of time indicators

(light) on circadian periodicity in humans. When equal periods of light-darkness alternation were in force, they observed the familiar pattern of pronounced, diurnally rhythmic fluctuations of catecholamines, for which amplitude was reduced under conditions of constant darkness.

Pituitary Hormones

Given the fact that the entry of light into the eye via the "energetic portion" of the visual pathway induces the hypothalamus and the

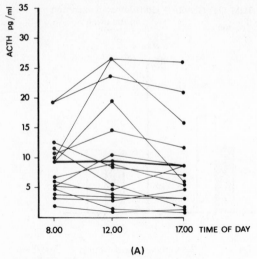

(A)

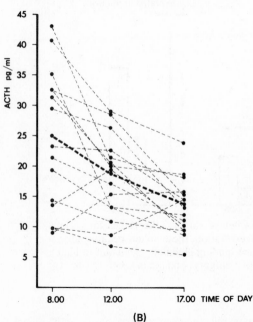

(B)

Fig. 56 A and B. ACTH blood levels in the blind (A) and normal sighted (B). The normal matutinal fall of plasma values is not present in the blind. An inverse behavior with rise of ACTH values is found in part. Solid line, individual curves (n = 15); solid line, average (Hollwich and Dieckhues).

pituitary (Scharrer 1937, 1964; Scharrer and Scharrer 1963; Hollwich 1948–1974; Hollwich and Tilgner 1961–1965; Hollwich and Dieckhues 1966–1975; Hollwich et al 1966–

1969, 1971, 1977), it follows that practically all secondary hormonal glands (for example, the adrenal cortex, thyroid, gonads) and possibly the pineal as well are influenced in a stimulatory and regulatory manner. If these photoimpulses are absent, as is the case with blind people, the question arises whether abnormalities in the secretion of the pituitary hormones ensue. In addition to existing biological methods, radioimmunological means have been developed recently which make it possible to measure even the slightest hormonal concentrations (e.g., ACTH). Diurnally rhythmic fluctuations have been found for numerous pituitary hormones, for example, ACTH (Ney et al 1963; Demura et al 1966; Berson and Yalow 1968; Krieger 1975), gonadotropins (Baker 1975), HGH (Krieger and Glick 1972; Plotnick et al 1975), and TSH (Odell and Odell 1965; Mertz and Isele 1964; de Costre 1971).

Studies of the growth hormone of the anterior lobe of the pituitary were conducted with 60 blind persons as compared to 25 with normal sight and with 20 cataract patients before (blind) and after (with sight) surgery (Hollwich 1973; Dieckhues 1974; Hollwich and Dieckhues 1975) (see Figs. 54 and 55). For the blind an average value of 1.16 pg/100 ml was found in comparison with 4.08 pg/100 ml for those with sight. Correspondingly, the values for cataract patients before surgery were 1.3 pg/100 ml; after surgery they were 2.52 pg/100 ml.

The individual daily curves were also found to be different in the blind; amplitude was lowered and diurnal average values were reduced ("neuroendocrine deficit").

Holding a central position in light stimulation via the eye-hypothalamus-pituitary-secondary hormonal glands system, ACTH also shows significant deviations when photostimulation via the eye is absent. Although less pronounced, diurnal fluctuations in the blind were similar to the findings for HGH. The ACTH content of the blood was lowered (Fig. 56A, B). Similar differences were also found for gonadotropin and TSH.

12
Natural Sunlight and Artificial Fluorescent Light

In the process of evolution all living creatures adapted to the natural alternation between daylight and darkness. Accordingly, it can be demonstrated that the systems of all organisms, from protozoa to man, are affected by the day-night sequence. Fluctuations occurring in the course of the day can deviate more than 100 percent from the diurnal mean value.

This natural daily rhythm was not interrupted until 1879 when Edison's invention of the incandescent lamp led to a completely new and different form of illumination. Subsequent research concentrated on producing the brightest light at the lowest cost without raising the question of whether this different kind of light might have a harmful effect on the human organism. Medical considerations were ignored as the "similarity to daylight" of artificial lighting was pointed out.

Yet, if natural daylight is compared to artificial light, important differences can be demonstrated regarding the intensity of illumination and the spectral composition and monotony of artificial light.

Intensity

It is well known that a great discrepancy exists between the intensity of natural light outdoors and artificial light indoors. Whereas up to 100,000 lux can be measured outdoors on bright summer days, a level of lighting intensity in an indoor work area exceeding 2,000 or 3,000 lux is unlikely.

A study by Range (1971) serves as an example of this. A work area was chosen outdoors where the incidence of light would not be affected by any obstruction. A test subject was seated at a desk facing north, i.e., in a direction that provided a maximum of uniform brightness. Test sheets with typewritten text and a computer punch card were placed in front of the volunteers. Both were to be judged successively according to their brightness. The test was given at different times of day, i.e., under differing conditions of light intensity. Fifty percent of the test subjects found the range from 2,800 to 4,250 lux to be an acceptable level of illumination.

The results show that the eye and the human organism adapted to these high levels of intense daylight out of doors without their being felt as noticeably disturbing. However, these same intensities in the form of artificial light would be found unacceptable to an extreme degree.

The unpleasant effect of high intensity artificial light comes from the stressful reaction elicited by increased metabolic activity. It must be emphasized here that the numerous effects of light on the human and animal organism that have been cited do not only produce a beneficial "natural stimulation" of the pituitary gland and the adrenal cortex; if the stimulus becomes too strong, they bring about an unspecific stress reaction.

Ever since Selye conducted his experiments, it has been known that stress of any kind leads to increased secretion of the adrenal cortex and that a build-up of stress factors or prolonged stress can result in the appearance of abnormalities and pathological changes in the organism. Therefore, the sensory influx of environmental stimuli can only be as much as can be accommodated by the regulatory systems. This influx must occur in physiological doses in order to keep the regulatory systems intact. On the other hand, an increase in the absorption of environmental influences via the sensory organs can lead to an overload in the regulatory system, thus causing pathological reactions in the organism.

Hollwich and Dieckhues (1966, 1968) studied eosinopenia in human blood after exposure to varying intensities of artificial light (see Fig. 29). The results indicate that as the intensity of the light increases, the eosinopenic effect occurs earlier and more markedly as a result of an increased secretion of cortisol from the adrenal cortex. Similar findings were reported by Radnot (1961). Tilgner (1967) even found a lineal dependence of eosinopenia on the logarithm of light intensity.

Even though the threshold for physiological stimulation by means of artificial light and for the pathological stress effect of light varies from person to person, still we should keep in mind that an increase in the intensity of light to 2,000 and 3,000 lux—sometimes called for by architects and lighting experts—can trigger a stress reaction in a relatively large number of people. In combination with our stress-laden surroundings, this can lead to pathological disturbances in the organism (due to so-called light pollution).

Spectral Differences

If the spectral composition of natural light (balance of brightness according to Harmon [1951]) is compared to that of artificial light, it is evident that sunlight evinces a continuous slight rise in the progression of high frequency wavelengths of light, reaching a maximum in the yellow-green area, then declining slightly until the infrared area. On the other hand, the artificial light of fluorescent lamps, which is of special interest because of its widespread use in interior lighting, does not show any continuity in the spectral distribution curve and is moreover broken up by the very intense mercury vapor lines at 406 nm, 436 nm, 546 nm, and 578 nm (Fig. 57). The disturbance in the spectral distribution curve in the case of fluorescent lamps is in part so pronounced that two or more maxima in varying wavelength areas appear. This difference in the spectral composition of artificial light causes a differing reaction in the organism, as Hollwich and Tilgner (1962) were able to prove by means of animal experiments. They irradiated five-month-old drakes with monochromatic light of differing wavelengths for a period of 21 days. The following results were attained: orange light enlarged the testicles six-fold and red light 16-fold when the reproductive cells were fully mature (see Fig. 48). Short-wave blue light, however, had no effect.

Thus, the stimulatory effect of light on the growth and maturation of the testicles is a function of specific wavelengths in the visible spectrum. It is significant in this regard that the development of the testicles is influenced by those wavelengths at the low fre-

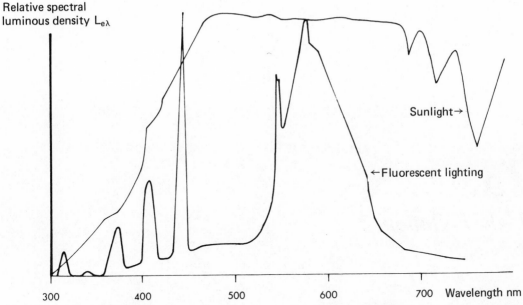

Fig. 57. Differences in the spectral composition of artificial light and sunlight. The chart shows the spectral distribution of luminous density in fluorescent lighting of one of the widely used tubes and sunlight. Sunlight: Continuous rise from short-wave ultraviolet light to green-yellow, then continuous fall to long-wave red light. Fluorescent light: According to the type of fluorescent tubes, there are differing amounts of the individual spectral colors. In addition, the continuity is broken by very intensive changing vapor lines at 406, 436, 546, and 577 nm. (In incandescent lighting there is the well-known larger amount of red light.)

quency end of the spectrum, an area of visible light which plays a subordinate role in the visual process.

The Monotony of Artificial Lighting

Whereas natural daylight is subject to continuous fluctuations in brightness and color because of cloud formation, sunrise, and twilight, artificial light evinces a monotony in brightness and color lasting from the moment the light is turned on until it is turned off. But we know from experience that for the biological regulatory mechanism to work properly, continuous variations in the amounts of stimulation are necessary to sustain its power to function. The adverse condition of permanent monotony carries with it the danger that this regulatory mechanism may be restricted in its role of governing the normal functions of the organism, thereby inducing pathological disturbances.

Until the present, problems with artificial lighting have been considered to be primarily technical, but it is now time to direct attention to the medical aspects. Man has adapted completely to natural daylight. Artificial light, which differs to a high degree from sunlight in its composition, should be regarded only as supplementary and not as a replacement of equal value. Above all in the case of children who attend schools without windows, we must be prepared for the eventual appearance of pathological consequences.

13
Light Pollution

Edison's invention of the carbon filament lamp in the year 1879 represented the beginning of a new era that replaced the pine torch and the wax candle. Work hours could be extended past twilight and into the night. Work performance and work capacity rose to a degree unheard of previously.

Since that time lighting experts have sought to heighten the intensity of lamps and decrease their heat emission, which results in cutting costs at the same time.

Today we live in the era of fluorescent lamps that can uniformly light every last corner of large and even extremely large spaces. The fluorescent lamps are installed as "bands of light" in the ceiling; they not only cast their light directly into the room but also onto the usually bright white ceiling and walls which reflect it back indirectly into the room. If the building is without windows or if daylight is excluded or seasonally lacking, then a thoroughly illuminated shadowless space is created which Höfling (1973) has aptly termed a "light cage." All objects in this space are brightly irradiated without any effect of depth and have a somewhat "incorporeal" appearance. Human skin takes on an unnatural sallow color, making,

for example, the faces of men or women look older.

As if it were not a fact that light involves the whole body, these bands of light in bright ceilings are found not only in public buildings, conference rooms, banks, offices, and factories, but in schools also. Not only is the adult exposed to this unnatural artificial flood of light but the growing child is as well. In addition, a minimum lighting intensity of from 1,000 to 1,200 lux is considered necessary in the child's workplace also.

In the winter months the child on schooldays as well as the worker in an office, store, or factory perceives artificial light not just during working hours but also on the public transportation used to get to and from school or work. During this time (with the exception of a few weekend hours) all functions of the human organism are exposed to an artificial photostimulus via the eye which is further heightened when the intense photostimulus of the television screen is added to it.

The most familiar result of this constant stimulus on the autonomic, i.e., unconscious nervous system is the increasing insomnia of the city dweller who is deprived of relaxation in the evening with the presently used light sources.

Wurtman, in the course of his investigations of the pineal organ with Axelrod, devoted special attention to the influence of light's entry into the eye on the organism. He wrote in 1969:

> For the past few generations, humans have spent much of their lives under artificial light sources, which often were designed to satisfy cosmetic considerations and whose spectra bear little similarity to the natural sunlight under which life on earth evolved. There are essentially no data to help us evaluate the biologic consequences of living under incandescent bulbs or standard "cool-white" fluorescent lights. If, in fact, excess exposure to artificial light sources or inadequate exposure to natural light has harmful biologic effects, we may find ourselves in a generation or two worrying about "light pollution." Someone ought to try to rule out this possibility now. (p. 37)

Nevertheless, artificial light without doubt has the capacity to increase performance. The inaccurate conclusion is often drawn, however, that this increase in performance is based solely on the improvement in visibility caused by the high intensity of illumination of from 2,000 to 3,000 lux. But light not only has the optic effect of improving vision: via the energetic portion of the optic pathway it also affects the entire organism, as previous chapters have discussed. Intense photostimulus causes increased secretion of ACTH and cortisol (see Chap. 12) and as a result, work performance increases during the first hours of exposure, only to decline sharply thereafter.

In this connection Hollwich et al (1977) studied the effects of intense artificial illumination on young voluntary subjects who were students. The results were that during two weeks of exposure to an intensity of 3,500 lux (fluorescent lamp "cool white") there was a continual rise in ACTH and cortisol excretion which reached stress levels. After a subsequent two-week return to natural daylight the "stress hormones" ACTH and cortisol returned to normal levels (Fig. 58).

These results also show that natural light, "the forgotten parameter" (Saltarelli 1977), is a basic element of vital processes. The extraterrestrial light emitted by the sun acts as an "energetic transmitter" via the "energetic portion" of the optic pathway (Hollwich 1948, see Fig. 58) for all living things. Entering the eye, it stimulates the hormonal glands and metabolic processes to act together harmoniously.

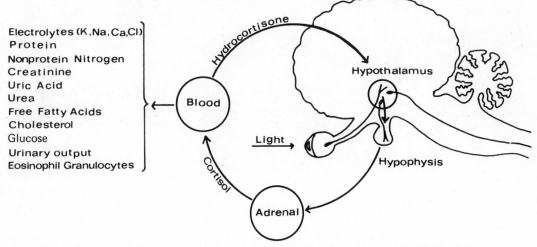

Fig. 58. Influence of light via the eye and the energetic portion of the optic pathway leading from the retina to the hypothalamus and the hypophysis on the endocrine-circle of function.

In order to avoid light pollution we should therefore utilize daylight as long as the season permits, both in schools and other places of work. If artificial illumination is necessary, it should be subject to variation by a stage-selector switch and should not exceed an average value of 500 lux for the school and 700 lux for the average place of work.

Artificial sources of light should approach the spectral range of natural light as closely as possible. There are two ways to reach this goal: first, as Meiners (1977) and Hollwich et al (1978) stated, by a combined form of light (fluorescent tubes and incandescent lamps) and, second, as Wurtman (1975) proposed, by a broad spectrum fluorescent lamp with a tube simulating sunlight in the visible and ultraviolet ranges. Recently we tested this tube and compared it under equal conditions with the standard cool-white fluorescent lamp (see Fig. 59) under the same stress-like intensity of 3,500 lux. With the broad spectrum tube we got a significantly less pronounced reaction of the "stress hormones" ACTH and cortisol than we found with one of the widely used standard cool-white lamps (Spectrum, see Fig. 57). In other words, from the standpoint of health, this broad spectrum tube is much better tolerated regarding the endocrine response of the human body than the standard cool-white one. We reported this result at the recent meeting of the International Commission of Illumination at Lausanne, Switzerland (Hollwich, July 1978).

14

The Importance of Light in Metabolism in Man and Animal: Summary

When we speak of the eye we generally think of its function as a camera whose sole task is to transmit to man the form, color, and brightness of the environment. The second and equally important function of the eye as a receptor for extravisual photostimuli is still generally unknown even today. The eye uses light not only as the medium of vision; light entering the eye regulates and stimulates numerous autonomic, i.e., unconscious metabolic and hormonal processes such as sugar balance, water balance, blood count, sexual function and much more, as has been discussed in detail in previous chapters.

Whereas numerous experiments with many animals (plaice, frog, duck, roebuck, etc.) have by now proved the influence upon them of light entering the eye, the influence of visually perceived light on the human organism, if mentioned at all, was until recently subject to doubt and regarded as unproven.

To investigate these questions, the author began experiments over thirty years ago (1947) on the blind (later also on the war blind) at the Eye Clinic and the Medical Clinic of the University of Munich, continuing these later with co-workers Tilgner in Jena (1961–1965) and Dieckhues in Münster (1966–1977). With the supplemental aid of comparative studies before and after surgery of patients who went temporarily blind from acquired opacities of the lenses of both eyes, it was possible to prove the effect of light entering the eye in an objective, scientific manner by means of metabolic and radioimmunological hormone experiments.

Removing the opaque lens restores light's entry into the eye and returns two functions to patients who were virtually blind before the operation: they regain their sight, and their autonomic centers (hypothalamus-pituitary-pineal) are stimulated by extravisual photostimuli. As a result, these individuals experience a revitalization which is also clearly expressed in their faces (see Fig. 16). Their happiness at their regained vision doubtless plays a role here too. But happy impressions or experiences have only a temporary effect on the psyche as well as on metabolism and endocrine glands. Thus, the permanent postoperative improvement in metabolic condition (see Fig. 22) can be attributed exclusively to the regained extravisual photostimuli.

Our experiments demonstrate without a doubt that from the earliest beginnings light from the sun has not only made the human individual's vision possible but has also stimulated and vitalized his metabolic and hormonal balance.

If light's entry into the eye is blocked (e.g., by blindness), then all metabolic and hormonal processes occur at a lower than normal level. There is abnormal adaptation to increased stresses as well as to the day-night rhythm.

As a result of our research, the laws of the state of Nordrhein-Westfalen (Federal Republic of Germany) have recognized this fact. In evaluating the degree of occupational disability caused by blindness, 30 additional positive points are granted if it can be proved by tests of blood chemistry that the lack of photostimulus has caused endocrine and metabolic abnormalities.

The time of the onset of blindness plays a role in determining the extent of these changes; becoming blind as a child causes much stronger side effects than if one becomes blind as an adult. Further, it should be noted that the totally blind person, as a result of the lack of visual stimuli, exhibits stronger side effects than the blind who still perceive light or possess slight vestigial vision.

In contrast to the blind person, the individual with intact vision thus possesses an additional source of energy as a result of light's entry into the eye. For this reason the working-hypothetical designation energetic portion (in contrast to "visual portion") was chosen by the author in 1948 for that part of the optic pathway that perceives the extravisual photostimuli and conducts them to the autonomic centers in the brain (hypothalamus-pituitary-pineal, see Fig. 10).

This energetic effect of light applies to the natural as well as artificial variety. Whereas before Edison's invention the eye was exposed for milennia only to natural light, for nearly 100 years now natural light has been increasingly supplemented or even replaced by artificial light.

In contrast to natural light, artificial light has an unnatural and hence unphysiological stimulatory effect; the greater the intensity of the light involved, the greater this effect. This is true in special measure for windowless working areas whose only source of light is fluorescent lamps in the form of bands of light. Unnecessarily high intensity of artificial light leads to stresslike changes of metabolic and endocrine parameters (Hollwich et al 1977) traceable in the blood chemistry, as we were able to demonstrate in our experiments (Fig. 59). In addition to this, adults who work in a so-called light cage (Höfling 1973) and whose autonomic nervous system is unstable by nature may undergo an increase in their symptoms.

The situation is completely different for the growing child who experiences all surrounding stimuli with particular intensity. For this reason schools should remain flexible, utilizing natural light as long and as often as possible, even if pedagogical aims should suffer a bit as a result, for example, by sometimes holding classes outdoors.

If artificial light is necessary in the darker months, the inadequate natural illumination should be supplemented as needed during the day with stage-selector switches and be fully replaced only in the evening.

As demonstrated in Chapter 5 (Light and Growth) the child is retarded in growth if light's entry into the eye is lacking. The effect of supplemental artificial light may in turn contribute, along with other factors such as higher protein intake, to the acceleration in growth which has been observed in recent decades in all northern countries.

Over and above this, the child's autonomic nervous system suffers to a heightened degree from the extravisual stimulus of artificial light of marked spectral deficiency (Fig. 57) including that from the television screen, as attentive observers believe can be demonstrated.

In conclusion, it must be stated that man is definitely a dual being, a creature of cul-

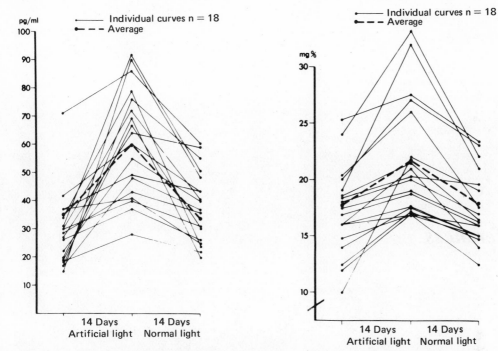

Fig. 59. ACTH (left) and cortisol (right) tests under artificial light (3,500 lux standard cool-white fluorescent lamp). Individual curves (uninterrupted line) of ACTH and cortisol as well as average curves (dotted line) for 18 subjects. Blood sample at 8 A.M. on an empty stomach under normal light (Test 1), after 2-week exposure to artificial light (Test 2), and after another two weeks of exposure to normal light (Test 3). The testing took place radioimmunologically. ACTH and cortisol increase significantly with artificial light (3,500 lux); after two weeks they reach stress levels that fall back to normal after subsequent exposure for two weeks to normal light.

ture as well as of nature. In conflict with the requirements and desires associated with his cultural self are his natural needs which call for activity (regular physical exercise out of doors) and good living habits (e.g., sufficient sleep before midnight), since these form the basis for the health of his organism.

Although human genius succeeded in imitating the light emitted by that "superterrestrial natural force, the sun" (Goethe), the imitation—necessary as it is for our civilization—is not a satisfactory substitute as far as our organism is concerned. Artificial sources of light are so-called "pseudo-suns" of culture. Natural light, involving the whole body, is a vital element like water and air. As such, it should accompany the human individual for as many hours of the day as the course of the seasons permits.

References

Alford, F. P., Baker, H. W. G., Burger, H. G.: The secretion rate of human growth hormone. I. Daily secretion rates, effect of posture and sleep. *J. Clin. Endocrinol. Metab.* **37**, 515, 1973.

Alford, F. P., Baker, H. W. G., Burger, H. G., et al: Temporal patterns of integrated plasma hormone levels. II. Follicle-stimulating hormone, luteinizing hormone, testosterone and estradiol. *J. Clin. Endocrinol. Metab.* **37**, 848, 1973.

Allen, M. B.: Effects of the exstirpation of the anterior lobe of the hypophysis of Rana pipiens. *Biol. Bull.* **32**, 163, 1917.

Anderson, J. A.: Thermo-variance spectrum in children. *Ann. N.Y. Acad. Sci.* **117**, 354, 1964.

Appel, W.: Über die Tagesschwankungen der Eosinophilen. *Z. Ges. Exp. Med.* **104**, 15, 1939.

Appel, W., and Hansen, K. J.: Lichteinwirkung, Tagesrhythmik der eosinophilen Leukozyten und Nebennierenrindensystem. *Dtsch. Arch. Klin. Med.* **199**, 530, 1952.

Armbruster, H., Vetter, W., Beckerhoff, R., et al: Diurnal variations of plasma aldosterone in supine man: relationship to plasma renin activity and plasma cortisol. *Acta Endocrinol. (Kbh.)* **80**, 95, 1975.

Aschner, B. (1929). "Handbuch der inneren Sekretion," Vol. II, 277. Verlag Curt Kabitzsch, Leipzig.

Aschoff, J.: Zeitgeber der tierischen Tagesperiodik. *Naturwiss.* **41**, 49, 1954.

Aschoff, J.: Der Tagesgang der Körpertemperatur beim Menschen. *Klin. Wschr.* **33**, 545, 1955a.

Aschoff, J.: Exogene und endogene Komponente der 24-Stunden-Periodik bei Tier und Mensch. *Naturwiss.* **42**, 569, 1955b.

Aschoff, J.: Tagesrhythmus des Menschen bei völliger Isolation. *Umschau* **66**, 378, 1966.

Aschoff, J. (1970). Circadiane Periodik als Grundlage des Schlaf-Wach-Rhythmus. *In* "Ermüdung, Schlaf und Traum. Hrsg. W. Baust." Bücher der Zeitschrift Naturwissenschaftliche Rundschau, Stuttgart.

Aschoff, J., Fatranska, M., Giedke, H.: Human circadian rhythms in continuous darkness: Entrainment by social cues. *Science* **171**, 213, 1971.

Aschoff, J., Pöppel, E., Wever, R.: Circadiane Periodik des Menschen unter dem Einfluss von Licht-Dunkel-Wechseln unterschiedlicher Periode. *Pflügers Arch.* **306**, 58, 1969.

Atkins, T. W., Bailey, C. J., Matty, A. J.: The effect of melatonin on insulin secretion in the rat and mouse. *J. Endocrin.* **58**, 17, 1973.

Axelrod, J.: Die Zirbeldrüse. *Endeavour* **29**, 144, 1970.

Axelrod, J., Wurtmann, R. J., Snyder, S. H.: Control of hydroxyndole-*O*-methyl-transferase activity in the rat pineal gland by environmental lighting. *J. Biol. Chem.* **240**, 949, 1965.

Axelrod, J., Wurtmann, R. J., Winget, C. M.: Melatonin synthesis in the hen pineal gland and its control by light. *Nature* **201**, 1134, 1964.

Baker, H. W. G.: Rhythms in the secretion of gonadotrophins and gonadal steroids. *J. Steroid Biochem.* **6**, 793, 1975.

Baker, J. R., and Rausom: Factors affecting the breeding of the field mouse (*Microtus agrestis*). Part 1. *Light. Proc. R. Soc. B* **110**, 313, 1932.

Balsam, A., Dobbs, C. R., Leppo, L. E.: Circadian variations in the concentration of plasma thyroxine and triidothonine in man. *J. Appl. Physiol.* **39**, 297, 1975.

Banting, F. G., and Best, Ch.: The internal secretion of the pancreas. *J. Labor and Clin. Med.* **7**, 251, 1922.

Barbarossa, C., et al: Attivita gonadotropa ipofisaria nel ratto privato di pineale. *Folia Endocr. (Pisa)* **12**, 535, 1959. *Zit. bei Kitay* 1967.

Barris, I.: Effect of experimental hypothalamic lesions upon blood sugar. *Am. J. Physiol.* **114**, 555, 1936.

Bar-sela, M. E., and Critchlow, V.: Delayed puberty following electrical stimulation of amygdalae in female rats. *Am. J. Physiol.* **211**, 1103, 1966.

Bartter, F. C., Delea, C. S., Halberg, F.: A map of blood and urinary changes related to circadian variations in adrenal cortical function in normal subjects. *Ann. N.Y. Acad. Sci.* **98**, 969, 1962.

Baschieri, L., De Luca, F., Cramarossa, L., et al: Modifications of thyroid activity by melatonin. *Experienta* **19**, 15, 1963.

Becher, H.: Über ein vegetatives, zentralnervöses Kerngebiet in der Netzhaut des Menschen und der Säugetiere. *Acta Neurovegetativa* **8**, 421, 1953.

Becher, H.: Über ein vegetatives Kerngebiet und neurosekretorische Leistungen der Ganglienzellen der Netzhaut. *Klin. Mbl. Augenheilk. Beih.* **23**, 1, 1955.

Belyaeva, T. I.: The influence of the duration of illumination on the development of the silkworm. *Zool. Z.* **18**, 407–411, 1939.

Benedict, F. G.: Studies in body temperature. I. Influence of the inversion of daily routine. The temperature of night workers. *Am. J. Physiol.* **11**, 145, 1904.

Benedict, F. G., and Snell, J. F.: Körpertemperaturschwankungen mit besonderer Rücksicht auf den Einfluss, welchen die Umkehrung der täglichen Lebensgewohnheit beim Menschen ausübt. *Pflügers Arch.* **90**, 33, 1902.

Benkö, E.: Weitere Angaben über die durch Lärmschäden bedingte Gesichtsfeldeinengung. *Ophthalmologica (Basel)* **138**, 449, 1959.

Benoit, J.: Activation sexuelle obtenue chez le canard par l'eclairment artificiel pendant la période de répos génital. *Compt. Rend. Acad. Sci.* **199**, 1671, 1934.

Benoit, J.: Rôle des yeux et de la voie nerveuse oculohypophysaire dans la gonadostimulation par la lumière artificielle chez le canard domestique. *Compt. Rend. Soc. Biol.* **129**, 231, 1938.

Benoit, J.: Action de la lumière visible, par l'intermédiaire de l'oeil, sur diverses fonctions de l'organisme des vertebrés, et en particulier sur la fonction de reproduction. *Scientia Ser. (Como)* **6**, 55, 1, 1961a.

Benoit, J.: Action de la lumière visible sur l'organisme, par l'intermédiaire de l'oeil et du système nerveux végétatif. *Bull. Soc. d'Ophthal.* **8**, 855, 1961b.

Benoit, J.: The role of the eye and of the hypothalamus in the photostimulation of gonads of the duck. *Ann. N.Y. Acad. Sci.* **117**, 204, 1964.

Benoit, J., and Assenmacher, I.: Le control hypothalamique de l'activité préhypophysaire gonadotrope. *F. Physiol. (Paris)* **47**, 427, 1955.

Benoit, J., Assenmacher, J., Brard, E.: Action d'un eclairment permanent prolongé sur l'évolution testiculaire du canard pekin. *Arch. Anat. Micr. Morph. Exp.* **48** (Suppl.), 5, 1959.

Benoit, J., Da Lage, Ch., Muel, B., Kordon, C., Assenmacher, J.: Localisation dans la spectre visible de la zone de sensibilité rétinienne maximale aux radiations lumineuses impliquées dans la gonadostimulation chez le canard pekin impubère. *C.R. Acad. Sci. Ser. D* **263**, 62, 1966.

Bergfeld, W.: Der Einfluss des Tageslichtes auf die Rattenschilddrüse mit Berücksichtigung des Grundumsatzes. *Endokrinologie* **6**, 269, 1930.

Bernard, Cl. (1885). "Leçons sur les Phénomènes

de la Vie, communs aux Anímaux et aux Végétaux." J. B. Baillière, Paris.

Berson, S. A., and Yalow, R. S.: Radioimmunoassay of ACTH in plasma. *J. Clin. Invest.* **47**, 2725, 1968.

Bissonette, T. H.: Studies on the sexual cycle in birds. Effects of light of different intensities upon the testis activity of the European starling. *Physiol. Zool.* **4**, 542, 1931.

Bissonette, T. H.: Modification of mammalian sexual cycles; reactions of ferrets *(Putorius vulgaris)* of both sexes to electric light added after dark in November and December. *Proc. Royal Soc. Biol.* **110**, 327, 1932.

Bissonette, T. H.: Inhibition of the stimulating effect of red light on testis activity in *Sturnus vulgaris* (starling) by a restricted diet. *Biol. Bull.* **65**, 452, 1933.

Bissonette, T. H.: Sexual photoperiodicity in the blue jay *(Cyanocitta cristata)*. *Wilson Bull.* **51**, 227, 1939.

Bissonette, T. H., and Wadlund, A. P. R.: Spermatogenesis in *Sturnus vulgaris* irrefractory period and acceleration in relation to wave length and rate of increase of light ration. *J. Morphol.* **52**, 403, 1951.

Bjerner, B., and Swensson, A.: Schichtarbeit und Rhythmus. *Acta Med. Scand. Suppl.* **278**, 102, 1954.

Bliss, E. L., Sandberg, A. A., Nelson, D. H., Kris, E. N.: The normal levels of 17-hydroxycorticosteroids in the peripheral blood of man. *J. Clin. Invest.* **32**, 818, 1953.

Bloch, S.: Versuche über den Einfluss intermittie-render Belichtung auf die Genitalfunktion der Maus. *Rev. Suisse Zool.* **71**, 687, 1964. *Rev. Suisse Zool.* **72**, 859–964, 1965.

Blümcke, S.: Zur Frage einer Nervenfaserverbindung zwischen Retina und Hypothalamus. *Z. Zellforsch.* **48**, 261, 1958.

Bodenheimer, S., Winter, J. S. D., Faiman, C.: Diurnal rhythms of serum gonadotropins, testosterone estradiol and cortisol in blind men. *J. Clin. Endocrinol. Metab.* **37**, 472, 1973.

Böhme, A.: Über die Schwankungen der Serumkonzentrationen beim gesunden Menschen. *Dtsch. Arch. Klin. Med.* **103**, 522, 1911.

Bouchardat: Du diabète sucré. Mém. de l'Académie de Médecine, 1851.

Bouma, P. I.: Farbe und Farbwahrnehmung. Eindhoven, 1951.

Braden, A. W. H.: The relationship between the diurnal light cycle and the time of ovulation in mice. *J. Exptl. Biol.* **34**, 177, 1957.

Brands, K. H.: Der Einfluss des Lichtes auf die Schilddrüsenfunktion der Maus. *Ärztl. Forsch.* **8**, 36, 1954.

Brednow, W. (1976). "Spiegel, Doppelspiegel und Spiegelungen—eine 'wunderliche Symbolik' Goethes. Sitzungsberichte der Sächsischen Akademie der Wissenschaften zu Leipzig, math.-naturwiss. Klasse, Bd. 112, Heft 1." Akademie-Verlag, Berlin (p. 12).

Bresnik, W., and Hohenegger, M.: Zur Tagesrhythmik der Kalzium- und Phosphorausscheidung im Harn bei Kranken mit Nykturie. *Wiener Z. Innere Med.* **48**, 361, 1967.

Breuer, H., Kaulhausen, H., Mühlbauer, W., Fritzsche, G., Vetter, H. (1974): Circadian rhythm of the renin–angiotensin–aldosterone system. *In* "Chronobiological Aspects of Endocrinology." Symposia Medica Hoechst, Stuttgart 1974.

Browman, L. G.: Light in its relation to activity and oestrus rhythmus in the albino rat. *J. Exp. Zool.* **75**, 375, 1937.

Brown, A., and Goodall, A. L.: Normal variations in blood haemoglobin concentration. *J. Physiol.* **104**, 404, 1946.

Brugsch, Th., Dresel, K., Lewy, F. H.: Stoffwechselneurologie der Medulla oblongata. *Verh. Dtsch. Ges. Inn. Med.* **32**, 144, 1920/21.

Büchner, H., and Kukla, D.: Die absolute Grösse der Sella turcica als Massstab für die Entwicklungsstufe der Hypophyse. *Klin. Mbl. Augenheilk.* **124**, 529, 1954.

Buddecke, E. (1971). "Grundriss der Biochemie," 2nd ed. W. de Gruyter, Berlin.

Bugnon, Cl., and Moreau, N.: Modifications cytologiques préhypophysaires chez le rat blanc épiphysectomisé ou soumis à l'action d'extraits acétoniques d'épiphyse de boeuf. *Ann. Sci. Univ. Besançon, Méd. Sér.* **2** (35), 37, 1961.

Buhl, H.: Schwankungen des Serumcholesterins am Tag und in der Nacht. *Münch. Med. Wschr.* **49**, 2490, 1966.

Bünning, E., and Joerrens, G.: Tagesperiodische antagonistische Schwankungen der Blauviolett-Gelbrot-Empfindlichkeit als Grundlage der photo-periodischen Diapause-Induktion bei Pieris brassicae. *Z. Naturforsch.* **15b**, 205–213, 1960.

Burger, J. W.: Some aspects of the roles of light intensity and daily length of exposure to light in the sexual photoperiodis activation of the male starling. *J. Exptl. Zool.* **81**, 33, 1939.

Burger, J. W.: Further studies on the relation of the daily exposure to light to the sexual activation of the male starling. *J. Exptl. Zool.* **84**, 350, 1940.

Burger, J. W.: On the relation of day length to the phases of testicular involution and inactivity of the spermatogenetic cycle of the starling. *J. Exptl. Zool.* **105**, 259, 1947.

Burger, J. W.: The effect of photic and psychic stimuli on the reproductive cycle of the male starling, *Sturnus vulgaris. J. Exptl. Zool.* **124**, 227, 1953.

Burger, J. W., Bissonette, T. H., Doolittle, H. D.: Some effects of flashing light on testicular activity in the male starling *(Sturnus vulgaris). J. Exptl. Zool.* **90**, 73, 1942.

Butenandt, O.: Humanes Wachstumshormon. *Beih. Z. Klin. Päd.* **72**, 1974.

Campbell, J. A., and Webster, T. A.: Day and night urine during complete rest, laboratory routine, light muscular work and oxygen administration. *J. Biochem.* **15**, 660, 1922a.

Campbell, J. A., and Webster, T. A.: Effect of severe muscular work on composition of the urine. Note on urinary tides and excretory rhythm. *J. Biochem.* **16**, 106, 507, 1922b.

Camus, J., and Roussy, G.: Experimental researches on the pituitary body. *Endocrinology* **4**, 507, 1920.

Camus, J., Gournay, J. J., Le Grand, A.: Lésions nerveuses et diabète sucré. *Paris Méd.* **13**, 267, 1923.

Carnicelli, A.: Effects of epiphysectomy on karyometry of hypothalamic nuclei in rats. *Folia Endocrin. (Pisa)* **16**, 229, 1963.

Carrel, A. (1932). "Der Mensch, das unbekannte Wesen." Dtsch. Verlagsanstalt, Stuttgart.

Chossat, C.: 1843 erstmals tagesschwankungen der körpertemperaturen an vögeln (tauben) nachgewiesen. *Memoires des Savants Étrangers.* **8**, 438, 1843.

Clark, J. H.: The action of light on the leucocyte count. *Am. J. Hyg.* **1**, 39, 1921.

Clarke, J. R., and Kennedy, J. P.: Effect of light and temperature upon gonad activity in the vole. *Gen. Comp. Endocrinol.* **8**, 474, 1967.

Clementi, F., De Virgilis, G., Mess, B.: Influence of pineal gland principles on gonadotropin-producing cells of the rat anterior pituitary gland: An electron-microscopy study. *J. Endocrinol.* **44**, 241, 1969.

Conroy, R. W. T. L., and Mills, J. N. (1970). "Human Circadian Rhythms." J. A. Churchill, London.

Costre de, P., Buhler, U., Degroot, L. J., Refetoff, S.: Diurnal rhythm in total serum thyroxine levels. *Metabolism* **20**, 782, 1971.

Cramer, H.: Neurohormonale Steuerung unter besonderer Berücksichtigung der Steuerung der Hypophysenfunktion bei Thyreotoxikosen, Basedow und Hyperfollikulinämie. *Med. Klin.* **47**, 1453, 1952.

Cramer, W., and Drew, A. H.: The effect of light on the organism. *Brit. J. Exp. Pathol.* **4**, 271, 1923.

Cremer, R. J., Perryman, P. W., Richards, D. H.: Influence of light on the hyperbilirubinaemia of infants. *Lancet* **1**, 1094, 1958.

Critchlow, V. (1963). The role of light in the neuroendocrine system. *In* "Advances in Neuroendocrinology" (A. V. Nalbandov, ed.), p. 372. Univ. of Illinois Press, Urbana, Ill.

Cropp, F.: Über den Einfluss schlechter kohlensäurereicher Luft sowie von Lichtabschluss auf wachsende Tiere. *Arch. f. Hyg.* **90**, 279, 1922.

Csaba, G., and Nagy, S. U.: The regulatory role of the pineal gland on the thyroid gland, adrenal medulla and the islets of Langerhans. *Acta Med. et Biol. Germ.* **31**, 617, 1973.

Csaba, G., Reti, I., Fischer, J.: Effect of the pineal body on the thyroid-thymus correlations. *Acta Med. Acad. Sci. Hung.* **27**, 183, 1970.

Czyba, J. C., Girod, C., Durand, N.: Sur l'antagonisme épiphyso-hypophysaire et les variations saisonnières de la spermatogénèse chez le hamster doré. *C.R. Soc. Biol.* **158** (1), 742, 1964.

Daane, T. A., and Parlow, A. F.: Serum FSH and LH in constant light-induced persistent estrus: Short term and long term studies. *Endocrinology* **88**, 964, 1971.

Dale, A., Berthelot, A., Boucher, D., Thieblot, L.: Valeurs de la thyréostimuline hypophysaire et des acides aminés iodés thyroidiens en fonction de l'eclairment chez la lapine adulte. *C.R. Soc. Biol. (Paris)* **166**, 1296, 1972.

D'Amour, M. C., and Keller, A. D.: Blood sugar studies following hypophysectomy and experimental lesions of hypothalamus. *Proc. Soc. Exp. Biol. Med.* **30**, 1175, 1933.

Dayton, G. D., Traber, W. J., Kaufmann, M. A., Gunter, L. M.: Overt behavior manifested in bilaterally patched patients. *Am. J. Ophthal.* **59**, 864–870, 1965.

Debeljuk, L.: Effect of melatonin on the gonadotrophic function of the male rat under constant illumination. *Endocrinology* **84**, 937, 1969.

DeLacerda, L., Kowarski, A., Johanson, A. J., Athanasiou, R., Migeon, C. J.: Integrated concentration and circadian variation of plasma testosterone in normal men. *J. Clin. Endocrinol. Metab.* **37**, 366, 1973.

DeLaet, M. H., Brion, J. P., LeCleroq, R., Virasoro, E., Copinsci, G.: Etudes des concentrations intégrées du cortisol et de l'hormone de croissance au cours du nycthémère chez l'homme normal. *Ann. d'Endocr.* **35**, 219, 1974.

Demura, H., West, C. O., Nugent, C. A., Nakagama, K., Tyler, F. H.: A sensitive radioimmunoassay for plasma ACTH levels. *J. Clin. Endocrinol.* **26**, 1297, 1966.

Descovich, G. C., Kühl, J. F. W., Halberg, F., et al: Age and catecholamine rhythms. *Chronobiologia* **1**, 163, 1973.

Desjardins, C., Ewing, L. L., Johnson, B. H.: Effects of light deprivation upon the spermatogenic and steroidogenic elements of hamster testis. *Endocrinology* **89**, 791, 1971.

Deuel, H. J., Butts, J. S., Hallman, L. F., Murray, S., Blunden, H.: Studies on ketosis. Diurnal changes in liver glykogen. *J. Biol. Chem.* **123**, 257, 1938.

Dieckhues, B.: Die Bedeutung der Lichtperzeption durch das Auge auf den Hormonhaushalt des Menschen. *Klin. Mbl. Augenheilk.* **165**, 291, 1974.

Djavid, I.: Über die Tagesschwankungen der Eosinophilenzahlen im Blut und die Beeinflussung der Eosinophilen durch Adrenalin. *Klin. Wschr.* **14**, 930, 1935.

Dobrowska, A., Rewkiewicz-dziarska, A., Szarska, I., Gill, J.: Seasonal changes in haematological parameters, level of serum proteins and glycoproteins, activity of the thyroid gland, suprarenals and kidneys in the common vole. *J. Interdiscipl. Cycle Res.* **5**, 347, 1974.

Dodt, E., and Heerd, E. J.: Mode of action of pineal nerve fibers in the frog. *J. Neurophysiol.* **25**, 405, 1962.

Doe, R. P., Flink, E. B., Goodsell, M. G.: Relationship of diurnal variation in 17-hydroxycorticosteroid levels in blood and urine eosinophils and electrolyte excretion. *J. Clin. Endocrinol.* **16**, 196, 1956.

Doering, C. H., Kraemer, H. C., Keith, H., Brodie, H., Hamburg, D. A.: A cycle of plasma testosterone in the human male. *J. Clin. Endocrinol.* **40**, 492–500, 1975.

Domarus, A. V.: Die Bedeutung der Kammerzählung der Eosinophilen für die Klinik. *Dtsch. Arch. f. Klin. Med.* **171**, 333, 1931.

Donovan, B. T., and Lockhart, A. N.: Light and the timing of ovulation in the guinea-pig. *J. Reprod. Fert.* **30** (2), 207–211, 1972.

Döring, G. K., Schaeffers, E., Weber, G.: Über die 24-Stunden-Rhythmik im Eiweissgehalt des Blutserums beim Menschen. *Pflügers Arch.* **253**, 165, 1951.

Dubois, M. R.: Sur la variation de résistance des mammifères hivernants à l'inanition. *C.R. Soc. Biol. (Paris)* **54**, 272, 1902.

Echave Llanos, J. M., Bade, E. G., Badran, A. F. (1967). Circadian rhythms in growth progress. *In* "The Cellular Aspects of Biorhythms" (H. v. Mayersbach, ed.), pp. 175–180. Springer, New York.

Elfvin, L. G., Petren, T., Sollberger, A.: Influence of some endogenous and exogenous factors on diurnal glycogen rhythms in chicken. *Acta Anat.* **25**, 286, 1955.

Ellendorf, F., and Smidt, D.: Der Einfluss unterschiedlicher Beleuchtung auf die neurosekretorische Aktivität, Pubertät und Sexualfunktion von Mäusen. *J. Neuro-visceral Relations* **10**, 220, 1971.

Elliott, J. A., Stetson, M. H., Menaker, M.: Regulation of testis function in golden hamsters: A circadian clock measures photoperiodic time. *Science* **178**, 771, 1972.

Emlen, S. T.: Bird migration: Influence of physiological state upon celestial orientation. *Science* **165**, 716, 1969.

Engelmann, W.: Phase shifting of eclosion in *Drosophila pseudoobscura* as a function of the energy of the light pulse. *Z. Vergl. Physiol.* **64**, 111–117, 1969.

Faiman, C., and Ryan, R. J.: Diurnal cycle in serum concentration of FSH in men. *Nature* **215**, 857, 1967.

Farkas, G. V.: Zur Pathologie der Bluteiweisskörper. *Z. Exp. Med.* **63**, 64, 1928.

Farrell, G.: Glomerulotropic activity of an acetone extract of pineal tissue. *Endocrinology* **65**, 239, 1959.

Farrell, G.: Adrenoglomerulotropin. *Circulation* **21**, 1009, 1960.

Farrell, G., Powers, D., Otani, T.: Inhibition of ovulation in the rabbit: Seasonal variation and effects of indoles. *Endocrinology* **83**, 599, 1968.

Fatranska, M.: Circadian rhythms of the urinary 17-OHCS and VMA in continuous light during sound and light deprivation. *J. Interdiscipl. Cycle Res.* **2**, 247, 1971.

Faure, J. M. A., Bensch, Cl., Vincent, J. D.: Influence de la lumière sur le comportement et sur la fonction ovarienne chez le lapin. *J. Neurovisceral Relations* **10**, 187, 1971.

Fendler, K.: The effect of illumination on the oxytocin content of the neurohypophysis and hypothalamus in the rat. *Acta Physiol. Hung.* **31** (2), 127–131, 1967.

Fisher, B., and Fisher, E. R.: Observations on the eosinophil count in man, a proposed test of adrenal cortical function. *Am. J. Med. Sci.* **221**, 121, 1951.

Fiske, V. M.: Effect of light on sexual maturation, estrous cycle and anterior pituitary of the rat. *Endocrinology* **29**, 187, 1941.

Fiske, V. M., Bryant, G. K., Putnam, J.: Effect of light on the weight of the pineal in the rat. *Endocrinology* **66**, 489, 1960.

Fiske, V. M., Bryant, G. K., Putnam, J.: Effect of light on the weight of the pineal organ in hypophysectomized, adrenalectomized or thiouracil-fed rats. *Endocrinology* **71**, 130, 1962.

Fiske, V. M., and Leeman, S. E.: Observations on adrenal rhythmicity and associated phenomena in the rat: Effect of light on adrenocortical function; maturation of the hypothalamic neurosecretory system in relation to adrenal secretion. *Ann. N.Y. Acad. Sci.* **117**, 231, 1964.

Flink, E. B., and Doe, R. P.: Effect of sudden time displacement by air travel on synchronization of adrenal function. *Proc. Soc. Exp. Biol.* **100**, 498, 1959.

Foa, C.: Hypertrophie des testicules et de la crête, après extirpation de la glande pinéale chez le coq. *Arch. Ital. Biol.* **57**, 233, 1912.

Forsgren, E.: Über die rhythmische Funktion der Leber und ihre Bedeutung für den Kohlehydratstoffwechsel bei Diabetes und für die Insulinbehandlung. *Klin. Wschr.* **8**, 110, 1929.

Forsgren, E. (1935). "Über die Rhythmik der Leberfunktion, des Stoffwechsels und des Schlafes." Gumpert, Götëborg.

Fox, W., and Dessauer, H. C.: Photoperiodic stimulation of appetite and growth in the male lizard, *Anolis caroliniensis. J. Exp. Zool.* **134**, 557–575, 1957.

Franks, R. C.: Diurnal variation of plasma 17-hydroxycorticosteroids in children. *J. Clin. Endocrinol.* **27**, 75, 1967.

Fraps, R. M.: Photoperiodism in the female domestic fowl. *Science* **123**, 767, 1959.

Fraschini, F., Mess, B., Martini, L.: Pineal gland, melatonin and the control of LH-secretion. *Endocrinology* **82**, 919, 1968.

Frehn, J. L., and Liu, C.-C.: Effects of tempera-ture, photoperiod and hibernation on the testes of golden hamsters. *J. Exp. Zool.* **174**, 317, 1970.

Frey, E.: Mitteilung über die Existenz eines hypothalamisch-optischen Bündels. Sitzungsber. II. *Internat. Neurol. Kongr., London 1935. Rev. Neurol.* **2**, 1935.

Frey, E.: Über die hypothalamische Optikuswurzel des Hundes. *Bull. d. Schweiz. Akad. Med. Wiss.* **7**, 115, 1951.

Frey, E.: Neue anatomische Ergebnisse zur Phylogenie der Sehfunktion. *Beih. Klin. Mbl. Augenheilk.* **23**, 1955.

Friederiszick, F. K., and Seitz, B.: Lichttherapie beim Neugeborenen-Ikterus. Klinische Ergebnisse. *Fortschr. Med.* **88**, 327, 1970.

Fubini, S.: Über den Einfluss des Lichtes auf die Kohlensäureproduktion bei den Batrachiern, nach Wegnahme der Lungen. *Moleschott's Untersuchungen zur Naturlehre des Menschen und der Tiere* **12**, 103, 1881.

Fuchs, J.: Vom Einfluss des Lichtreizes auf den Stoffwechsel. *Dtsch. Med. Wschr.* **78**, 1054, 1953.

Fuchs, J.: Der blinde Harfner. *Ther. Ber.* **37**, 40, 1965.

Ganong, W. F., Shepherd, M. D., Wall, J. R., Van Brun, T. E. E., Clegg, M. T.: Penetration of light into the brain of mammals. *Endocrinology* **72**, 962, 1963.

Garot, L.: Les rayons ultra-violets modifient-ils la pression sanguine? *C.R. Biol.* **68**, 871, 1928.

Gaston, S., and Menaker, M.: Photoperiodic control of hamster testis. *Science* **158**, 925, 1967.

Geller, I.: Ethanol preference in the rat as a function of photoperiod. *Science* **173**, 456, 1971.

Georgi, F.: Psycho-physische Korrelationen. I. Die Tagesrhythmik des Cholesterinspiegels bei endogenen Psychosen. *Schweiz. Med. Wschr.* **74**, 539, 1944.

Gerritzen, F.: Der 24-Stunden-Rhythmus in der Diurese. *Dtsch. Med. Wschr.* **64**, 746, 1938.

Gerritzen, F.: The diurnal rhythm in water, chloride, sodium and potassium excretion during a rapid displacement from east to west and vice versa. *Aerospace Med.* **33**, 697, 1962.

Gerritzen, F.: Influence of light on human circadian rhythms. *Aerospace Med.* **37**, 66, 1966.

Giedke, H., and Fatranska, M.: Tagesperiodik der Rectaltemperatur sowie der Ausscheidung von Elektrolyten, Katecholaminmetaboliten und 17-Hydroxy-Corticosteroiden mit dem Harn beim Menschen mit und ohne Lichtzeitgeber. *Int. Arch. Arbeitsmed.* **32**, 43, 1974.

Gigon, A.: Licht und Kohlenhydratstoffwechsel. *Schweiz. Med. Wschr.* **34**, 859, 1929.

Gigon, A.: Biologische Lichtwirkung. *Klin. Wschr.* **42**, 1947, 1930.

Goldeck, H., Herrnring, G., Richter, U.: Die 24-Stunden-Periodik der Thrombozyten. *Dtsch. Med. Wschr.* **75**, 702, 1950.

Graffenberger, L.: Versuche über die Veränderungen, welche der Abschluss des Lichtes in der chemischen Zusammensetzung des tierischen Organismus und dessen N-Umsatz hervorruft. *Pflügers Arch.* **53**, 238, 1893.

Greving, R.: Beiträge zur Anatomie des Zwischenhirns und seiner Funktion, der anatomische Verlauf eines Faserbündels des N. opticus beim Menschen (Tr. supraoptico-thalamicus), zugleich ein Beitrag zur Anatomie des unteren Thalamusstiels. *Graefes Arch.* **115**, 523, 1925.

Grim, C., Winnacker, J., Peters, T., Gilbert, G.: Low renin, normal aldosterone and hypertension: Circadian rhythms of renin, aldosterone, cortisol and growth hormone. *J. Clin. Endocrinol. Metab.* **39**, 247, 1974.

Grober, I., and Sempell, O.: Die blutzusammensetzung bei jahrelanger Entziehung des Sonnenlichtes. *Dtsch. Arch. Klin. Med.* **129**, 305, 1919.

Groebbels, F. (1932). Der Vogel. I. Atmungswelt und Nahrungswelt. Berlin.

Gunderson, E. K. E.: Psychische Probleme in der Antarktis *Dtsch. Ärztblatt* **66**, 1010, 1969.

Häberlein, C., Kestner, O., Lehmann, F. Wilbrand, E., Georges, B.: Die Heilwirkung des Nordseeklimas. *Klin. Wschr.* **2**, 2020, 1923.

Halberg, F.: Some physiological and clinical aspects of 24-hour periodicity. *Lancet* **73**, 20, 1953.

Halberg, F.: Zeitgeber. *Acta Med. Scand.* **307**, 117, 1955.

Halberg, F.: When to treat. *Indian J. Cancer* **12**, 1, 1975.

Halberg, F., Albrecht, P. G., Barnum, C. P.: Phase shifting of liver-glycogen in intact mice. *Am. J. Physiol.* **199**, 400, 1960.

Halberg, F., French, L. A., Gully, R. J.: 24-hour rhythm in rectal temperature and blood eosinophils after hemidecortication in human subjects. *J. Appl. Physiol.* **12**, 381, 1958.

Halberg, F., and Ulstrom, R. A.: Morning changes in number of circulating eosinophils in infants. *Proc. Soc. Exp. Biol. Med.* **80**, 747, 1952.

Halberg, F., and Vissher, M. B.: Regular diurnal physiological variation in eosinophil levels in five stocks of mice. *Proc. Soc. Exp. Biol. Med.* **75**, 846, 1950.

Halberg, F., Vissher, M. B., Bittner, J. J.: Eosinophil rhythm in mice: Occurrence, effects of illumination, feeding and adrenalectomy. *Am. J. Physiol.* **174**, 109, 1953.

Halberg, F., Vissher, M. B., Bittner, J. J.: Relation of visual factors to eosinophil rhythm in mice. *Am. J. Physiol.* **179**, 229, 1954.

Halberg, F., Zander, H. A., Houglum, M. W., Mühlemann, H. R.: Daily variations in tissue mitosis, blood eosinophils and rectal temperature of rats. *Am. J. Physiol.* **177**, 361, 1954.

Hammond, J. (1973). Seasonal changes of pelt, body weight and gonadal activity in the ferret, and the influence of photoperiod in their regulation. *In* "Int. Congress: The Sun in the Service of Mankind," B 17. Unesco-House, Paris.

Harmon, D. B. (1951). "The Co-ordinated Classroom." American Seating Company, Grand Rapids, Michigan.

Hartwig, H. G.: Electron microscopic evidence for a retinohypothalamic projection to the suprachiasmatic nucleus of Passer domesticus. *Cell Tiss. Res.* **153**, 89, 1974.

Hauff, J. (1941). Über den 24-Stunden-Rhythmus menschlicher Körperfunktionen, insbesondere der Leberfunktion, der Urinausscheidung und des Blutwassergehaltes. Inaug. Diss. (M.D. Thesis), Tübingen.

Hayhow, W. R.: An experimental study of the accessory optic fiber system in the rat. *J. Comp. Neurol.* **113**, 281, 1959.

Hayhow, W. R., Webb, C., Jervie, A.: The accessory optic fiber system in the rat. *J. Comp. Neurol.* **115**, 187, 1960.

Hecht, K., Treptow, K., Poppel, M., Hecht, T.: Zur Abhängigkeit pharmakologischer Effekte von der Umgebungshelligkeit. *Acta Biol. Med. Germ.* **20**, 757, 1968.

Heilmeyer, L. (1942). "Handbuch der Inneren Medizin," p. 47. Springer, Berlin.

Hellbrügge, Th.: The development of circadian rhythms in infants. *Cold Spring Harbor Symp. Quant. Biol.* **25**, 311, 1960.

Hellbrügge, Th.: Entwicklung der Tag-Nacht-Periodik im Kindesalter. *Wiss. Z. Humboldt. Univ. Berlin Math. Naturw. R.* **14**, 263, 1965.

Hellmann, L., Nakada, F., Curti, J., et al: Cortisol is secreted episodically by normal man. *J. Clin. Endocrinol.* **30**, 411, 1970.

Hendrickson, A., Wilson, M. E., Toyne, M. J.: The distribution of optic nerve fibers in *Macaca mulatta*. *Brain Res.* **23**, 425, 1970.

Hendrickson, A. E., Wagoner, N., Cowan, W. M.: An autoradiographic and electron microscopic study of retino-hypothalamic connections. *Z. Zellforsch.* **135**, 1, 1972.

Herbert, J. (1971). The role of the pineal gland in the control by light of the reproductive cycle of the ferret. *In* "The Pineal Gland" (G. W. Wolstenholme and J. Knight, eds.), a Ciba Foundation Symposium.

Hermann, L., and Fuchs, R. F. (1914). "Handbuch der vergleichenden Physiologie III."

Heubner, O.: Tumor der Glandula pinealis. *Dtsch. Med. Wschr.* (Vereinsbeilage, Nr. 29) **24**, 214, 1898.

Hildebrandt, G.: Störungen biologischer Rhythmik. *Umweltmedizin* **7**, 152, 1973.

Himwich and Keller (1933). Cited in F. Hollwich (1950).

Hipkin, L. J.: Gonadotrophin inhibitory properties of pineal extracts. *Nature* **228**, 1202, 1970.

Hobert, H.: Über Blutregeneration anaemisierter Mäuse im Dunkeln, im Licht und unter Einwirkung künstlicher Höhensonne. *Klin. Wschr.* **2**, 1213, 1923.

Hoffmann, J. C.: Effects of light deprivation on the rat estrous cycle. *Neuroendocrinology* **2**, 1–10, 1967.

Höfling, G. (1973). "Kopfschmerzen durch Leuchtstofflampen? ('Neonlicht'). Untersuchungen und Vorschläge eines Augenarztes," p. 63. Schilling-Verlag, Herne.

Hofmann-Credner, D.: Die beeinflussung der wasserdiurese beim menschen durch flackerlicht. *Helvet. Med. Acta* **20**, 1, 1953.

Hogben, L. T.: Studies on the pituitary. I. The melanophore stimulant in posterior lobe extracts. *Biochem. J.* **16**, 16–23, 1922.

Hogben, L. T.: The pigmentary effector system. IV.: A further contribution to the role of pituitary secretion in amphibian color response. *Brit. J. Exper. Biol.* **1**, 75, 1924.

Hogben, L. T.: Some observations on the production of excitement pallor in reptiles. *Transact. Roy. Soc. S. Africa* **16**, 1928.

Hollwich, F.: Untersuchungen über die Beeinflussung funktioneller Abläufe, insbesondere des Wasserhaushaltes durch energetische Anteile der Sehbahn. *Ber. Dtsch. Ophthal. Ges. Heidelberg* **54**, 326, 1948.

Hollwich, F.: Untersuchungen über die Beeinflussung funktioneller Abläufe, insbesondere des Wasserhaushaltes durch energetische Anteile der Sehbahn. *Graefes Arch. Ophthal.* **149**, 592, 1949.

Hollwich, F.: Untersuchungen über die funktionellen Beziehungen zwischen dem energetischen Anteil der Sehbahn und dem Zuckerhaushalt. *Graefes Arch. Ophthal.* **150**, 529, 1950.

Hollwich, F.: Zwischenhirn-Hypophysensystem und Sella turcica. *Ber. Dtsch. Ophthal. Ges. Heidelberg* **57**, 173, 1951.

Hollwich, F.: Experimentelle Untersuchungen über die Beziehungen des "energetischen Anteils der Sehbahn" zu der Regeneration des Blutes. *Münch. Med. Wschr.* **95**, 212, 1953.

Hollwich, F.: Die Bedeutung von Lichtimpulsen für den Zuckerstoffwechsel. *Acta Neuroveg.* **9**, 330, 1954.

Hollwich, F.: Der Einfluss des Augenlichtes auf die Regulation des Stoffwechsels. *In* Auge und Zwischenhirn. 23. *Beih. Klin. Mbl. Augenheilk.* **5**, 95, 1955.

Hollwich, F.: Der Einfluss des Lichtes über das Auge auf den Farbwechsel des Frosches. *Klin. Mbl. Augenheilk* **133**, 784, 1958.

Hollwich, F.: Der Lichteinfluss über das Auge als Stimulans hormoneller Vorgänge. *Med. Klinik* **58**, 1914, 1963.

Hollwich, F.: Auge und Vegetativum. *Studium Generale* **17**, 752, 1964a.

Hollwich, F.: The influence of light via the eyes on animals and man. *Ann. N. Y. Acad. Sci.* **117**, 105, 1964b.

Hollwich, F.: Augenlicht und hypothalamo-hypophysäres System. *Ver. Dtsch. Ges. Inn. Med.* **71**, 278, 1965.

Hollwich, F.: Augenlicht und vegetative Funktionen. *Nova Acta Leopoldina* **31**, 189, 1966.

Hollwich, F.: Der Einfluss des Augenlichtes auf Stoffwechselvorgänge. *Acta Neuroveg.* **30**, 201, 1967.

Hollwich, F. (1973). Influence of light on metabolism. *In* "Int. Congress: The Sun in the Service of Mankind," B 35, pp. 1–10. Unesco-House, Paris.

Hollwich, F. (1974). Biological effects of solar radiation on man. Effects on the eye. *In* "Progress in Biometeorology" (S. W. Tromp, ed.), p. 373. Swets & Zeitlinger, Amsterdam.

Hollwich, F., and Dieckhues, B.: Der einfluss des Lichtes auf die Eosinophiliereaktion bei sehenden und blinden Personen. *Klin. Mbl. Augenheilk.* **149**, 840, 1966.

Hollwich, F., and Dieckhues, B.: Augenlicht und Nebennierenrindenfunktion. *Dtsch. Med. Wschr.* **92**, 2335, 1967a.

Hollwich, F., and Dieckhues, B.: Der Einfluss des Augenlichtes auf den Kohlenhydratstoffwechsel. *Med. Klinik* **62**, 748, 1967b.

Hollwich, F., and Dieckhues, B.: Eosinopenie-
reaktion und Sehvermögen. *Klin. Mbl. Augenheilk.* **152**, 11, 1968.

Hollwich, F., and Dieckhues, B.: Augenlicht und
Hormonhaushalt. *Z. Physik. Med.* **2**, 485,
1971a.

Hollwich, F., and Dieckhues, B.: Endokrines
System und Erblindung. *Dtsch. Med. Wschr.*
96, 363, 1971b.

Hollwich, F., and Dieckhues, B.: Endocrine system and blindness. *Ger. Med. Month.* **1**, 122,
1971c.

Hollwich, F., and Dieckhues, B.: Circadian
rhythm in the blind. *J. Interdiscipl. Cycle Res.*
2, 291, 1971d.

Hollwich, F., and Dieckhues, B. (1972a). Circadian rhythm of cortisol level in normal subjects and in the blind. *In* "Contemporary Ophthalmology" (J. G. Bellows, ed.). Williams &
Wilkins, Baltimore.

Hollwich, F., and Dieckhues, B.: Thrombozyten-
Tagesrhythmik und Augenlicht. *Klin. Mbl.
Augenheilk.* **160**, 60, 1972b.

Hollwich, F., and Dieckhues, B.: Die Wirkung
von Tages- und Kunstlicht auf den tierischen
und menschlichen Organismus. *Fortschr.
Med.* **90**, 25, 1972c.

Hollwich, F., and Dieckhues, B.: Augenlicht und
Blutbild. *Nova Acta Leopoldina* **38**, 299, 1973.

Hollwich, F., and Dieckhues, B.: Augenlicht und
Leberstoffwechsel. *Klin, Mbl. Augenheilk.*
164, 449, 1974a.

Hollwich, F., and Dieckhues, B. (1974b).
Changes in the circadian rhythm of blind people. *In* "Chronobiology" (L. Scheving et al,
eds.). G. Thieme, Stuttgart.

Hollwich, F., and Dieckhues, B.: Augenlicht und
Biorhythmus. Internat. Kongr. "Rhythmische
Funktionen in biologischen Systemen." Vi-
enna, September 1975.

Hollwich, F., Dieckhues, B., Jünemann, G.: Ein-
fluss der okularen Lichtperzeption auf die
Azetonitrilletalität weisser Mäuse. *Klin. Mbl.
Augenheilk.* **149**, 539, 1966.

Hollwich, F., Dieckhues, B., Jünemann, G.:
Über den Einfluss des Lichtes auf den endo-
genen Fettstoffwechsel. *Symp. Dtsch. Ges.
Endokrinologie* **12**, 223, 1967.

Hollwich, F., Dieckhues, B., Meiners, C. O.:
Kann Tageslicht durch kuenstliche Beleuchtung ersetzt werden? *Glasforum* **1**, 2, 1978.

Hollwich, F., Dieckhues, B., Schrameyer, B.:
Die physiologische Bedeutung des Lichtes für
den Menschen. *Licht-Technik* **27**, 388, 1975.

Hollwich, F., Dieckhues, B., Schrameyer, B.:
Die Wirkung des natürlichen und künstlichen
Lichtes über das Auge auf den Hormon- und
Stoffwechselhaushalt des Menschen. *Klin.
Mbl. Augenheilk.* **171**, 98–104, 1977.

Hollwich, F., Fatranska, M., Dieckhues, B.: Der
Einfluss der Lichtaufnahme durch das Auge
auf den Tagesrhythmus der 3-Methoxy-4-Hy-
droxy-Mandelsäure-Ausscheidung. *Klin. Mbl.
Augenheilk.* **155**, 895, 1969.

Hollwich, F., Niermann, H., Dieckhues, B.: Der
Einfluss des Augenlichtes auf den Gonadotro-
pingehalt des Serums beim Menschen. *Extrait
d'Arch. D'Anat., d'Hist., d'Embryol.* **51**, 335,
1968.

Hollwich, F., Niermann, H., Dieckhues, B.: Einfluss des Augenlichtes auf die Sexualsteuerung
bei Mensch und Tier. *J. Neurovisc. Relations
Suppl.* **10**, 247, 1971.

Hollwich, F., and Tilgner, S.: Experimentelle
Untersuchungen über den Einfluss monochro-
matischen Lichtes auf die Hodenentwicklung
des Erpels. *Klin. Mbl. Augenheilk.* **139**, 828,
1961a.

Hollwich, F., and Tilgner, S.: Experimentelle
Untersuchungen über den photosexuellen Re-
flex (réflexe opto-sexuel) bei der Ente.
Ophthalmologica **142**, 572, 1961b.

Hollwich, F., and Tilgner, S.: Der Einfluss der
Lichtwirkung über das Auge auf Schilddrüse
und Hoden. *Dtsch. Med. Wschr.* **87**, 2674,
1962.

Hollwich, F., and Tilgner, S.: Über die gonadotrope und thyreotrope Wirkung der Bestrahlung des Auges mit monochromatischem
Licht. *Endokrinologie* **44**, 167, 1963a.

Hollwich, F., and Tilgner, S.: Das Verhalten der
Eosinophilenzahl als Indikator der okularen
Lichtreizwirkung. *Klin. Mbl. Augenheilk.*
142, 531, 1963b.

Hollwich, F., and Tilgner, S.: Über den Einfluss
des Lichts auf die Entblutungsanaemie von
Ratten und Mäsen. *Med. Klinik.* **59**, 85, 1964a.

Hollwich, F., and Tilgner, S.: Reaktionen der
Eosinophilenzahl auf okulare Lichtreize.
Dtsch. Med. Wschr. **89**, 1430, 1964b.

Hollwich, F., and Tilgner, S.: Changes in the eosinophil count in response to ocular stimulation by light. *Ger. Med. Month.* **10**, 14, 1965.

Holmgren, N.: *Ark. Zool.* **2**, 1, 1918.

Homma, K., Wilson, W. O., Siopes, T. D.: Eyes
have a role in photoperiodic control of sexual
activity of coturnix. *Science* **178**, 421, 1972.

Hönig, M., Wallner, E., Radnot, M.: Verhalten

der endogenen Eosinopenie bei Erkrankungen des Sehnerven. *Acta Chir. Acad. Sci. Hung.* **5**, 113, 1964.

Hörmann, G.: Über die Ursachen der Tagesschwankungen der Temperatur des Menschen. *Z. Biol.* **36**, 319, 1898.

Hosemann, H.: Unterliegt der Menstruationszyklus der Frau und die tägliche Geburtenzahl solaren und lunaren Einflüssen? *Dtsch. Med. Wschr.* **24**, 815, 1950.

Hübener, H. J., Kreuziger, H., Heintz, R., Koch, M.: Flammenphotometrische Bestimmungen der tagesrhythmischen Ausscheidung von Natrium und Kalium beim Menschen. *Z. Ges. Exp. Med.* **119**, 523, 1952.

Hunt, R.: The influence of thyroid feeding upon poisoning by acetonitrile. *J. Biol. Chem.* **1**, 33, 1905–1906.

Isachsen, L.: Blut und Sonnenstrahlung. Zit. bei Kestner. *Fortschr. d. Therapie* **12**, 390–392, 1925.

Ishibashi, T., Hahn, D. W., Srivasta, L., Kumaresan, P., Turner, C. W.: Effect of pinealectomy melatonin on feed consumption and thyroid hormone secretion rate. *Proc. Soc. Exptl. Biol. Med.* **122**, 644, 1966.

Jafarey, N. A., Khan, M. Y., Jafarey, S. N.: Role of artificial lighting in decreasing the age of menarche. *Lancet* **2**, 471, 1970.

"Jahrbuch Geflügelwirtschaft." (1973). Verlag Eugen Ulmer, Stuttgart.

Januszkiewicz, W., and Wocial, B.: Recent data on noradrenalin. *Pol. Arch. Med. Wewnet.* **30**, 207, 1960.

Jarrett, R. J. (1974). Diurnal variation in glucose tolerance; associated changes in plasma insulin, growth hormone and non-esterified fatty acids and insulin sensitivity. *In* "Chronobiological Aspects of Endocrinology" (J. Aschoff, F. Ceresa, F. Halberg, eds.). G. Thieme, Stuttgart.

Jefferson, J. M.: A study of the subcortical connections of the optic tract system of the ferret, with special reference to gonadal activation by retinal stimulation. *J. Anat.* **75**, 106, 1940.

Jendralski, H.-J.: Heilung eines Falles von Diabetes insipidus nach doppelseitiger Kataraktextraktion. *Klin. Mbl. Augenheilk.* **118**, 319, 1951.

Jöchle, W.: Experimentelle Untersuchungen zur neuroendokrinen Steuerung der Mauser beim Haushuhn. *Symp. Dtsch. Ges. Endokrinologie* **8**, 416, 1962.

Jöchle, W.: Umwelteinflüsse auf neuroendokrine

Regulationen: Wirkungen langfristiger, permanenter Beleuchtung auf jugendliche und erwachsene Ratten. *Zbl. Vet. Med.* **10**, 654, 1963.

Johansson, J. E.: Über die Tagesschwankungen des Stoffwechsels und der Körpertemperatur im nüchternen Zustande und vollständiger mu-Skelruhe. *Skand. Arch. Physiol.* **8**, 85, 1898.

Jores, A.: Die Urineinschränkung in der Nacht. *Dtsch. Arch. Med.* **175**, 224, 1933.

Jores, A.: Die 24-Stundenperioden des Menschen. *Med. Klinik.* **30**, 468, 1934a.

Jores, A.: Über den Einfluss des Lichtes auf die 24-Stundenperiodik des Menschen. *Dtsch. Arch. Klin. Med.* **176**, 544, 1934b.

Jores, A.: Nykturie als Symptom zentral-nervöser Störungen. *Klin. Wschr.* **13**, 130–132, 1934c.

Jores, A.: Physiologie und Pathologie der 24-Stunden-Rhythmik des Menschen. *Erg. Inn. Med. u. Kinderheilk.* **48**, 574, 1935a.

Jores, A.: Änderungen des Hormongehaltes der Hypophyse mit dem Wechsel von Licht und Dunkelheit. *Klin. Wschr.* **14**, 1713, 1935b.

Jores, A.: Endokrines und vegetatives System in ihrer Bedeutung für die Tagesperiodik. *Dtsch. Med. Wschr.* **64**, 989, 1938.

Judd, H. L., Parker, D. C., Rakoff, J. S., Hopper, B. R., Yen, S. S.: Elucidation of mechanisms of the nocturnal rise of testosterone in men. *J. Clin. Endocrinol. Metab.* **38**, 134, 1974.

Jundell, J.: Über die nycthemeralen Temperaturschwankungen im ersten Lebensjahr des Menschen. *Jb. Kinderheilk.* **59**, 521, 1904.

Jürgensen, Th. (1873). Die Körperwärme des gesunden Menschen. Leipzig.

Kaiser, I. H., and Halberg, F.: Circadian aspects of birth. *Ann. N.Y. Acad. Sci.* **98**, 1056–1068, 1962.

Kalich, J.: Wissenschaftliche Untersuchungen im Dienste der modernen "Hühnerfarm." *Umschau* **62**, 741, 1962.

Kaloud, H.: Zur somatischen Entwicklung und Motorik blinder Kinder. *Wiener Med. Wschr.* **120**, 895, 1970.

Kapen, S., Boyar, R. M., Finkelstein, J. W., Hellmann, L., Weitzman, E. D.: Effect of sleep-wake cycle reversal on luteinizing hormone secretory patterns in puberty. *J. Clin. Endocrinol. Metab.* **39**, 293, 1974.

Kappers, J. A.: The development, topographical relations and innervation of the epiphysis cerebri in the albino rat. *Z. Zellforsch.* **52**, 163, 1960.

Kappers, J. A. (1965). Survey of the innervation of the epiphysis cerebri and the accessory pineal organs of vertebrates. *In* "Structure and Function of the Epiphysis Cerebri" (J. A. Kappers and J. P. Schade, eds.), Progress in Brain Research, Vol. 10, p. 87. Elsevier, Amsterdam.

Kappers, J. A.: The mammalian epiphysis cerebri as a center of neurovegetative regulation. *Acta Neuroveg.* **30**, 190, 1967.

Kappers, J. A.: The mammalian pineal organ. *J. Neurovisc. Rel. Suppl.* **9**, 140, 1969.

Kappers, J. A.: Regulation of reproductive system by the pineal gland and dependence on light. *J. Neuro-Visceral Relations* Suppl. X, 141, 1971.

Kappers, J. A., Smith, A. R., De Vries, R. A. C.: The mammalian pineal gland and its control of hypothalamic activity. *Prog. Brain Res.* **41**, 149, 1974.

Kärki, N. T.: The urinary excretion of noradrenaline and adrenaline in different age groups: Its diurnal variation and the effect of muscular work on it. *Acta Physiol. Scand.* **39** (Suppl. 132), 1–96, 1956.

Karlsson, J. O., and Sjöstrand, J.: Synthesis, migration and turnover of protein in retinal ganglion cells. *J. Neurochem.* **18**, 749, 1971.

Katz, F. H., Romfh, P., Smith, J. A.: Episodic secretion of aldosterone in supine man, relationship to cortisol. *J. Clin. Endocrinol. Metab.* **35**, 178, 1972.

Katz, F. H., Romfh, P., Smith, J. A.: Diurnal variation of plasma aldosterone, cortical and renin activity in supine man. *J. Clin. Endocrinol. Metab.* **40**, 125, 1975.

Katz, G., and Leffkowitz, M.: Die Blutkörperchensenkung. *Erg. Inn. Med.* **33**, 266, 1928.

Kaulhausen, H., Mühlbauer, W., Breuer, H.: Circadianer Rhythmus der Reninaktivität im Plasma des Menschen. *Klin. Wschr.* **52**, 631, 1974.

Kelly, D. E.: Pineal organs: Photoreception, secretion and development. *Am. Scient.* **50**, 597–625, 1962.

Kerenyi, N. A., and von Westarp, C.: Postnatal transformation of the pineal gland: effect of constant darkness. *Endocrinology* **88**, 1077, 1971.

Kestner, O.: Klimatologische Studien. Der wirksame Anteil des höhenklimas. *Z. Biol.* **73**, 1, 1921.

Kestner, O.: Blut und Sonnenbestrahlung. *Fortschr. Ther.* **1**, 390, 1925.

Kienast, B.: Über den Genitalcyclus bei blinden Frauen. Dissertation, Univ.-Frauenklinik Münster, 1955.

Kinson, G. A., and Peat, F.: The influences of illumination, melatonin and pinealectomy on testicular function in the rat. *Life Sci.* **10** (I)/5, 259, 1971.

Kinson, G. A., and Robinson, S.: Gonadal function of immature male rats subjected to light restriction, melatonin administration and removal of the pineal gland. *J. Endocrinol.* **47**, 391, 1970.

Kinson, G., and Singer, B.: The pineal gland and the adrenal response to sodium deficiency in the rat. *Neuroendocrinology* **2**, 283, 1967.

Kinson, G. A., and Singer, B. (1971). *In* "The Pineal Gland" (G. E. W. Wolstenholme and J. Knight, eds.), a Ciba Foundation Symposium, p. 274. Edinburgh, London.

Kitay, J. I.: Possible functions of the pineal gland. *Neuroendocrinology* **2**, 641, 1967.

Kitay, J. I., and Altschulte, M. D. (1954). "The Pineal Gland." Harvard Univ. Press, Cambridge, Mass.

Klein, D. C., and Weller, J. L.: Indole metabolism in the pineal gland: A circadian rhythm in N-acetyltransferase. *Science* **169**, 1093, 1970.

Klein, D. C., and Weller, J. L.: Rapid light-induced decrease in pineal serotonin N-acetyltransferase activity. *Science* **177**, 532, 1972.

Kleitman, N. (1939). "Sleep and Wakefulness as Alternating Phases in the Cycle of Existence." Univ. of Chicago Press, Chicago.

Kleitman, N., and Engelmann, Th.: Sleep characteristics of infants. *J. Appl. Physiol.* **6**, 269, 1953.

Kleitman, N., Titelbaum, S., Hoffmann, H.: The establishment of the diurnal temperature cycle. *Am. J. Physiol.* **119**, 48, 1937.

Knaus, H. (1950). "Physiologie Der Zeugung." Springer, Berlin.

Knoche, H.: Die Verbindung der Retina mit den vegetativen Zentren des Zwischenhirns und der Hypophyse. *Verh. Anat. Ges. Stockholm* **103**, 140, 1956.

Knoche, H.: Die retino-hypothalamische Bahn von Mensch, Hund und Kaninchen. *Z. Mikro-Anat. Forsch.* **63**, 461, 1957.

Knoche, H.: Neue Befunde über die Existenz einer retinohypothalamischen Bahn. *Verh. Anat. Ges. Zürich* **106/107**, 212, 1959.

Knoche, H.: Ursprung, Verlauf und Endigung der retinohypothalamischen Bahn. *Z. Zellforsch.* **51**, 658, 1960.

Köbberling, J., and Von Zurmühlen, A.: The circadian rhythm of free cortisol determined by urine sampling at two-hour intervals in normal subjects and in patients with severe obesity or Cushing's syndrome. *J. Clin. Endocrinol. Metab.* **38**, 313, 1974.

Kobryner, A.: Über den physiologischen Verlauf der Leukozyten beim Menschen. *Z. Klin. Med.* **102**, 470, 1926.

Koe, K. F., Höfler, W., Lüders, K.: Mittlere Hauttemperaturen und periphere Extremitätentemperaturen bei den tagesperiodischen Änderungen der Wärmeabgabe. *Arch. Physik. Ther.* **20**, 221, 1968.

Koenigsfeld, H.: Stoffwechsel und Blutuntersuchungen bei Bestrahlung mit künstlicher Höhensonne. *Z. f. Klin. Med.* **91**, 159, 1921.

Koleszar, G.: Endogene Eosinopenie als Index der retinalen Komponente. *Klin. Mbl. Augenheilk.* **152**, 510, 1968.

Kolpakov, M. G., Kolaeva, S. G., Polyak, M. G. (1974). Endogenous mechanisms for the synchronization of corticosteroid production and seasonal rhythms in hibernating animals. *In* "Chronobiology" (L. Scheving et al, eds.), p. 136. G. Thieme, Stuttgart.

König, A., and Meyer, A.: The effect of continuous illumination on the circadian rhythm of the antidiuretic activity of the rat pineal. *J. Interdiscipl. Cycle Res.* **2**, 255, 1971.

Kowarski, A., Lacerda, L., Migeon, C. J.: Integrated concentration of plasma aldosterone in normal subjects: Correlation with cortisol. *J. Clin. Endocrinol. Metab.* **40**, 205, 1975.

Kowarski, A., Thompson, R. G., Migeon, C. J., Blizzard, R. M.: Determination of integrated plasma concentration and true secretion rates of human growth hormone. *J. Clin. Endocrinol. Metab.* **32**, 356, 1971.

Kranzfeld, B.: Zur frage über die physiologischen Tagesschwankungen der Thrombozytenzahl. *Pflügers Arch.* **210**, 583, 1925.

Kraus, Fr. (1919). "Die allgemeine und spezielle Pathologie der Person. Klinische Syzygiologie," pp. 270 ff. and 275 f. G. Thieme, Leipzig.

Kresbach, E., and Rabel, Ch.: Zur Regulation der eosinophilen Leukozyten. *Wien. Klin. Wschr.* **66**, 295, 1954.

Kriebel, J.: Circadiane Periodik der Catecholamine beim Menschen. *Naturwissenschaften* **57**, 500, 1970.

Krieger, D. T.: Rhythms of ACTH and corticosteroid secretion in health and disease, and their experimental modification. *J. Steroid Biochem.* **6**, 785, 1975.

Krieger, D. T., Allen, W., Rizzo, F., Krieger, H. P.: Characterization of the normal pattern of plasma corticosteroid levels. *J. Clin. Endocrinol.* **32**, 266, 1971.

Krieger, D. T., and Glick, S. M.: Growth hormone and cortisol responsiveness in Cushing's syndrome: Relation to a possible central nervous system etiology. *Am. J. Med.* **52**, 25–40, 1972.

Krieger, D. T., Kreuzer, J., Rizzo, F. A.: Constant light: Effect on circadian pattern and phase reversal of steroid and electrolyte levels in man. *J. Clin. Endocrinol.* **29**, 1634, 1969.

Krieger, D. T., and Krieger, H. P.: Circadian pattern of plasma 17-hydroxycorticosteroid alteration by anticholinergic agents. *Science* **155**, 1421, 1967.

Kriens, O.: Untersuchungen über die absolute Eosinophilenzahl des kindlichen Blutes und ihr Verhalten nach Flickerlicht-Beleuchtung beider Augen. *Inaug. Diss. Med. Fak. Univ., Münster*, 1956.

Küchler, W.: Jahreszyklische Veränderungen im histologischen Bau der Vogelschilddrüse. *J. Ornithol.* **83**, 414, 1935.

Kühnau, J. (1971). Hormonale Regulationen unter Beteiligung des Pinealorgans. *In* "Handb. Allg. Path.," Vol. VIII, pp. 1, 197. Springer, Berlin.

Labhart, A. (1971). "Klinik der Inneren Sekretion," 2nd ed. Springer, Berlin.

LaFontaine, E., Ghata, J., LaVernge, J., et al: Rythmes biologiques et décalages horaires. *Concour Médical* **89**, 3731, 1967.

LaGoguey, M., Dray, F., Chauffournier, J. M., Reinberg, A.: Circadian and circannual rhythms of urine testosterone and epitestosterone glucuronides in healthy adult men. *Int. J. Chronobiol.* **1**, 91–93, 1973.

Lakatua, D. J., Haus, E., Gold, E. M., Halberg, F. (1974a). Circadian rhythm of ACTH and growth hormone in human blood; time relations to adrenocortical (blood and urinary) rhythms. *In* "Chronobiology" (L. Scheving, ed.), p. 123. G. Thieme, Stuttgart.

Lakatua, D. J., Haus, E., Halberg, F. (1974b). Habitual circadian timing of growth hormone (STH), adrenocorticotrophic hormone (ACTH), insulin, cortisol and glucose in human serum. *In* "Chronobiological Aspects of Endocrinology" (J. Aschoff, F. Ceresa, F. Halberg, eds.), p. 185. G. Thieme, Stuttgart.

Landau, J., and Feldman, S.: Diminished endogenous morning eosinopenia in blind subjects. *Acta Endocrinol.* **15**, 53, 1954.

Lang, K.: Über die Tagesschwankung in dem Schwefel—und Tryptophangehalt der menschlichen Serumeiweisskörper. *Arch. Exp. Path. Pharmak.* **154**, 337, 1930.

Lange, F.: Die Haltungsschäden und die Leibesübungen. *Münch. Med. Wschr.* **74**, 265, 1927.

Langerhans: Beiträge zur mikroskopischen Anatomie der Bauchspeicheldrüse. Diss., Berlin, 1869.

Laquer, F.: Untersuchungen der Gesamtblutmenge im Hochgebirge mit der griesbachschen Kongorotmethode. *Klin. Wschr.* **3**, 7, 1924.

Laurens, H., and Sooy, J. W.: The effect of light and of darkness on blood cell number of growing Albino rat. *Proc. Soc. Exp. Biol. Med.* **22**, 114, 1924.

Lenau, H., Hollwich, F., Dieckhues, B., Niermann, H.: Der Einfluss des Augenlichtes auf das männliche Keimdrüsenhormon. *Fortschritte der Fertilitätsforschung* **3**, 136–139, 1976.

Lerner, A. B., Case, F. D., Heinzelmann, R. V.: *J. Am. Chem. Soc.* **80**, 2587, 1958.

Leschke, E.: Klinische und experimentelle Untersuchungen über Diabetes insipidus, seine Beziehungen zur Hypophyse und zum Zwischenhirn. *Z. Klin. Med.* **86**, 201, 1918.

Lestradet, H., Deschamps, I., Giron, B. (1974). Diurnal variations of insulin in normal children. *In* "Chronobiological Aspects of Endocrinology" (J. Aschoff, F. Ceresa, F. Halberg, eds.), p. 239. G. Thieme, Stuttgart.

Levine, L., Taylor, D., Halberg, F.: Circadian rhythms before and after removal of both eyes for bilateral retinoblastoma. *Alb. Graefes Arch. Ophthal.* **188**, 263, 1973.

Levy, F. M., and Conge, G.: Action de la lumière sur l'éosinophilie sanguine chez l'homme. *C.R. Soc. Biol.* **147**, 586, 1953.

Lewis, P. R., and Lobban, M. C.: Persistence of 24 hr pattern in human subjects living on a 22 hr day. *J. Physiol.* **125**, 34P, 1954.

Lewis, P. R., Lobban, M. C., Shaw, T. J.: Patterns of urine flow in human subjects during a prolonged period of light on a 22 hour day. *J. Physiol.* **133**, 659, 1956.

Leyendecker, G., and Saxena, B. B.: Tagesschwankung von FSH und LH im menschlichen Plasma. *Klin. Wschr.* **48**, 236, 1970.

Liebe, S., and Keller, J.: Untersuchungen über die Akzeleration blinder Kinder. *Münch. Med. Wschr.* **107**, 264, 1965.

Liebermeister, C. (1875). "Handbuch der Pathologie und Therapie des Fiebers." G. Thieme, Leipzig.

Lincoln, G. A., Rowe, P. H., Racey, R. A. (1974). The circadian rhythm in plasma testosterone concentration in man. *In* "Chronobiological Aspects of Endocrinology" (J. Aschoff, F. Ceresa, F. Halberg, eds.), p. 137. G. Thieme, Stuttgart.

Lisk, R. D., and Kannwischer, L. R.: Light: Evidence for its direct effect on hypothalamic neurons. *Science* **146**, 272, 1964.

Lister, M. (1885). Reference in article by H. Winterstein in "Handbuch vergleichende Physiologie" (R. F. Fuchs, ed.), Vol. III (1, 2). Verlag G. Fischer, Jena, 1914.

Lobban, M. C.: The entrainment of circadian rhythms in man. *Cold Spring Harbor Symp. Quant. Biol.* **25**, 325, 1960.

Lobban, M. C.: Human renal diurnal rhythms in an arctic mining community. *J. Physiol.* **165**, 75, 1963.

Lobban, M. C. (1965). Dissociation in human rhythmic functions. *In* "Circadian Clocks" (J. Aschoff, ed.), p. 219. North-Holland, Amsterdam.

Lobban, M. C.: Daily rhythms of renal excretion in arctic-dwelling Indians and Eskimos. *Quart. J. Exp. Physiol.* **52**, 401, 1967.

Lobban, M. C.: Human renal diurnal rhythms at the equator. *J. Physiol.* **204**, 133, 1969.

Lobban, M. C.: Circadian rhythms of renal excretion in human subjects at different latitudes. *J. Interdiscipl. Cycle Res.* **2**, 273, 1971.

Lobban, M. C.: Human daily rhythms of renal excretion in a modern arctic indian settlement during the midwinter darkness. *J. Interdiscipl. Cycle Res.* **3**, 245, 1972.

Lobban, M. C.: Seasonal variations in daily patterns of renal excretion in modern Eskimo children. *J. Interdiscipl. Cycle Res.* **5**, 295, 1974.

Lobban, M. C., and Tredre, B. E.: Renal diurnal rhythms in blind subjects. *J. Physiol.* **170**, 29, 1964.

Lobban, M. C., and Tredre, B. E.: Perception of light and the maintenance of human renal diurnal rhythms. *J. Physiol.* **189**, 32P, 1967.

Luce-Clausen, E. M., and Brown, E. F.: The use of isolated radiation in experiments with the rat. *J. Nutr.* **18**, 551, 1939.

Lyman, C. P.: Control of coat colour in the varying hare. *Bull. Mus. Comp. Zool. Harvard* **93**, 393, 1943.

Lynch, H. J., Ozaki, Y., Shakal, D., Wurtman, R. J.: Melatonin excretion of man and rats: Effect of time of day, sleep, pinealectomy and food consumption. *Int. J. Biometeor.* **19**, 267–279, 1975.

MacFarlane, W. V. (1974). Seasonal cycles of human conception. *In* "Progress in Biometeorology" (S. W. Tromp, ed.), Div. A, Vol. 1, pp. 557–577. Swets & Zeitlinger, Amsterdam.

Magee, K., Basinska, J., Quarrington, B., Stanger, H. C.: Blindness and menarche. *Life Sci.* **9**, 7, 1970.

Malek, J., Gleich, J., Maly, V.: Characteristics of the daily rhythm of menstruation and labor. *Ann. N.Y. Acad. Sci.* **98**, 1042–1055, 1962a.

Malek, J., Suk, K., Brestak, M., Maly, V.: Daily rhythm of leucocytes, blood pressure, pulse rate, and temperature during pregnancy. *Ann. N.Y. Acad. Sci.* **98**, 1018, 1962b.

Manchester, R. C.: The diurnal rhythm in water and mineral exchange. *J. Clin. Invest.* **12**, 995, 1933.

Marshal, F. H. A.: The experimental modification of the oestrous cycle in the ferret by different intensities of light radiation and other methods. *J. Exp. Biol.* **17**, 139, 1940.

Marshal, F. H. A., and Bowden, F. P.: The effect of irradiation with different wave-lengths on the estrous cycle of the ferret, with remarks on the factors controlling sexual periodicity. *J. Exp. Biol.* **11**, 409, 1934.

Marti, A.: Wie wirken die chemischen Hautreize und Belichtung auf die Bildung der roten Blutkörperchen? *Verh. Dtsch. Ges. Inn. Med.* **15**, 598, 1897.

Martini, L. (1974). Circadian rhythm and the role of the pineal gland. *In* "Chronobiological Aspects of Endocrinology" (J. Aschoff, F. Ceresa, F. Halberg, eds.), p. 385. G. Thieme, Stuttgart.

Martini, L., Fraschini, F., Motta, M. (1968). Neural control of anterior pituitary functions. *In* "Recent Progress in Hormone Research" (E. D. Astwood, ed.), Vol. 24 (Peptide Hormones), p. 439. Academic Press, New York.

Marx, H. (1941). "Innere Sekretion—Handbuch der Inneren Medizin," Vol. VI. Springer, Berlin.

Marx, H.: Hypophysäre Insuffizienz bei Lichtmangel. *Klin. Wschr.* **24/25**, 18, 1946.

Mast, S. O.: Changes in shade, color and pattern in fishes and their bearing on the problems of adaptation and behaviour, with special reference to the flounders. *Bull. U.S. Bur. Fish.* **34**, 177–238, 1916.

Mayerson, H. S., Gunther, L., Laurens, H.: The physiological action of darkness, daylight and of carbon arc radiation. I. The effects of darkness on metabolism in the dog. *Am. J. Physiol.* **75**, 399, 1926a.

Mayerson, H. S., Gunther, L., Laurens, H.: The physiological action of darkness, daylight and carbon arc radiation. II. The effect of carbon arc radiation on metabolism in the dog. *Am. J. Physiol.* **75**, 421, 1926b.

McCord, C. P., and Allen, F. P.: *J. Exp. Zool.* **23**, 207, 1917.

Mehner, A. (1962). "Lehrbuch der Geflügelzucht: Züchtung, Fütterung und Haltung von Hühnern und Puten." Parey Verlag, Hamburg.

Meiners, C. O.: Der Architekt muss umlernen. *Dtsch. Architekten-u.-Ing.-Z.* **15**, 11, 1977.

Menaker, M., and Keatts, H.: Extraretinal light perception in the sparrow. II. Photoperiodic stimulation of testis growth. *Proc. Nat. Acad. Sci. USA* **60**, 146, 1968.

Menzel, W.: Über den heutigen Stand der Rhythmenlehre in Bezug auf die Medizin. *Z. Altersforsch.* **6** (26), 104, 1932.

Menzel, W.: Wellenlänge und Phasenlage der menschlichen Nierenrhythmik mit analysen nach dem blumeschen Verfahren. *Z. Ges. Exp. Med.* **116**, 237, 1950.

Menzel, W. (1962). "Menschliche Tag-Nacht-Rhythmik und Schichtarbeit." Benno Schwabe, Basel/Stuttgart.

Mering, J. v., and Minkowski, O.: Über Diabetes mellitus nach Pankreasexstirpation. *Schmiedebergs Arch.* **26**, 371, 1889.

Mertz, D. P., and Isele, W.: Tagesperiodische Änderungen der Dynamik des endogenen Jodstoffwechsels. *Med. Klin.* **59**, 1536, 1964.

Migeon, C. J., Tyler, F. H., Mahoney, J. P., et al: The diurnal variation of plasma levels and urinary excretion of 17-OHCS in normal subjects, night workers and blind subjects. *J. Clin. Endocrinol.* **16**, 622, 1956.

Milcu, I., Nanu-Ionescu, L., Marcean, R., Ionescu, V.: Diabetic cortisone-induced state and adrenalectomy in pinealectomized or pinealin treated rats. *Rev. Roum. Endocrinol.* **10**, 339, 1973.

Miles, A. L., and Laurens, H.: The physiological action of darkness, daylight and carbon arc radiation. III. The effects of darkness on some of the physical changes of the blood of dogs. *Am. J. Physiol.* **75**, 1926a.

Miles, A. L., and Laurens, H.: The physiological action of darkness, daylight and carbon arc radiation. IV. The effects of carbon arc radiation on some of the physical characters of the blood of dogs. *Am. J. Physiol.* **75**, 462, 1926b.

Milin, R.: Die wirkung des Lichtes auf den Hypophysenhinterlappen der Ratte. *Verh. Anat. Ges. Freiburg* **104**, 191, 1957.

Milin, R., and Ciglar, M.: Die Wirkung der Dunkelheit auf den Hypophysenhinterlappen. *Verh. Anat. Ges. Stockholm* **103**, 189, 1956.

Miline, R.: Influence de la lumière sur la structure de la glande thyroide. *Med. Pregl.* **13**, 1, 1952.

Mills, J. N.: Circadian rhythms during and after three months in solitude underground. *J. Physiol.* **174**, 217, 1964.

Mills, J. N., and Stanbury, S. W.: Persistent 24-hour renal excretory rhythm on a 12-hour cycle of activity. *J. Physiol.* **117**, 22, 1952.

Mills, J. N., and Thomas, S.: Diurnal excretory rhythms in a subject changing from night to day work. *J. Physiol.* **137**, 65, 1957.

Mindermann, H.: Die Bedeutung des Auges für Vegetativum und Psyche und seine Beteiligung an psychosomatischen Erkrankungen. *Inaug. Diss.* Mainz 1971.

Moleschott, J.: Über den Einfluss des Lichtes auf die Menge der vom Tierkörper ausgeschiedenen Kohlensäure. *Wiener Med. Wschr.* **43**, 1855.

Moore, R. Y.: Pineal response to light: Mediation by the accessory optic system in the monkey. *Nature* **222**, 781, 1969.

Moore, R. Y.: Retinohypothalamic projection in mammals: A comparative study. *Brain Res.* **49**, 403, 1973.

Moore, R. Y., Heller, A., Bhathagar, R. K., Wurtman, R. J., Axelrod, J.: Central control of the pineal gland: Visual pathways. *Arch. Neurol.* **18**, 208, 1968.

Moore, R. Y., and Lenn, N. J.: A retinohypothalamic projection in the rat. *J. Comp. Neurol.* **146**, 1, 1972.

Morgan, L. O., Vonderahe, A. R., Malone, E. F.: Pathological changes in the hypothalamus in diabetes mellitus. *J. Nerv. Dis.* **85**, 125, 1937.

Morin, L. P.: Ovulatory and body weight response of the hamster to constant light or pinealectomy. *Neuroendocrinology* **12**, 192, 1973.

Moszkowska, A. (1965). Structure and function of the epiphysis cerebri. *In* "Progress in Brain Research" (J. A. Kappers and J. P. Schade, eds.), p. 564. Elsevier, Amsterdam.

Moszkowska, A., Kordon, C., Ebels, J. (1971). Biochemical fractions and mechanisms involved in the pineal modulation of pituitary gonadotropin release. *In* "The Pineal Gland" (G. E. W. Wolstenholem and J. Knight, eds.), a Ciba Foundation Symposium.

Moszkowska, A., and Scemana, A.: L'épiphysectomie et la réponse photosexuelle du rat. *Arch. Anat.* **51**, 473, 1968.

Müller, H. J.: Die Saisonformenbildung von Araschnia levana, ein photoperiodisch gesteuerter Diapause-Effekt. *Naturwissenschaften* **42**, 134–135, 1955.

Müller, H. J.: Die Wirkung verschiedener diurnaler Licht-Dunkel-Relationen auf die Saisonformenbildung von Araschina levana. *Naturwissenschaften* **43**, 503–504, 1956.

Mullin, F. J.: Development of the diurnal temperature and motility patterns in a baby. *Am. J. Physiol.* **126**, 589P, 1939.

Narang, G. D., Singh, D. V., Turner, C. W.: Effect of melatonin on thyroid hormone secretion rate and feed consumption of female rats. *Proc. Soc. Exptl. Biol. Med.* **125**, 184, 1967.

Neal, Ch., Smith, C., Dubowski, K., Naughton, J.: 3-Methoxy-4-hydroxy-mandelic acid excretion during physical exercise. *J. Appl. Physiol.* **24**, 619, 1968.

Nelson, W., and Halberg, F.: An evaluation of time-dependent changes in susceptibility of mice to pentobarbital injection. *Neuropharmacology* **12**, 509, 1973.

Ney, R. L., Shimizu, N., Nicholson, W. E., Island, D., Liddle, G. W.: Correlation of plasma ACTH concentration with adrenocortical response in normal human subjects, surgical patients and patients with Cushing's disease. *J. Clin. Invest.* **42**, 1669, 1963.

Nicoloff, J. T.: A new method for the measurement of thyroidal iodine release in man. *J. Clin. Invest.* **49**, 1912, 1970.

Nieschlag, E. (1974). Circadian rhythm of plasma testoterone. *In* "Chronobiological Aspects of Endocrinology" (J. Aschoff, F. Ceresa, F. Halberg, eds.), p. 117. G. Thieme, Stuttgart.

Nitschkoff, St., and Kriwizkaja, G.: Lärmbelastung, akustischer Reiz und neurovegetative

Störungen, eine morpho-physiologische Studie. *Edition Leipzig* **22**, 153, 1968.

Norn, M.: Untersuchungen über das Verhalten des Kaliums im Organismus. II. Über Schwankungen der Kalium-, Natrium- und Chloridaus-scheidung durch die Niere im Laufe des Tages. *Skand. Arch. Physiol.* **55**, 184, 1929.

O'Connor, J. F., Wu, G. Y., Gallagher, T. F., Hellman, L.: The 24-hour plasma thyroxin profile in normal men. *J. Clin. Endocrinol. Metab.* **39**, 765, 1974.

Odell, W., and Odell, P.: Radioimmunoassay of thyrotropin in human serum. *J. Clin. Endocrinol.* **25**, 1179, 1965.

Oltramare, J. H.: Quelques réflexions à propos de l'action de l'obscurité sur les êtres vivants. *Soc. Biol.* **82**, 190, 1919.

Ortavant, R. (1973). Influence des radiations solaires thermiques et lumineuses sur l'activité sexuelle des mammifères domestiques. *In* "Int. Congress: "The Sun in the Service of Mankind," B 18. Unesco-House, Paris.

Ortavant, R., Mauleon, P., Thibault, C.: Photoperiodic control of gonadal and hypophyseal activity in domestic mammals. *Ann. N.Y. Acad. Sci.* **117**, 157–193, 1964.

Orth, D. N., and Island, D. P.: Light synchronization of circadian rhythm in plasma cortisol (17-OHCS) concentration in man. *J. Clin. Endocrinol.* **29**, 479, 1969.

Orth, D. N., Island, D. P., Liddle, G. W.: Experimental alteration of the circadian rhythm in plasma cortisol (17-OHCS) concentration in man. *J. Clin. Endocrinol.* **27**, 549, 1967.

Osterman, P. O., Wallin, G., Wide, L.: Nocturnal secretory patterns of FSH, LH and TSH. *Upsala J. Med. Sci.* **79**, 55, 1974.

Ott, J. N.: Some responses of plants and animals to variations in wavelights of light energy. *Ann. N.Y. Acad. Sci.* **117**, 624–635, 1964.

Parkes, A. S. (1968). Seasonal variation in human sexual activity. *In* "Genetic and Environmental Influences on Behaviour" (J. M. Thoday and A. D. Parkes, eds.), p. 128. Oliver & Boyd, Edinburgh.

Parmelee, A. H.: A study on one infant from birth to eight months of age. *Acta Paediatr.* **50**, 160, 1961.

Patkai, P.: Interindividual differences in diurnal variations in alertness, performance and adrenaline excretion. *Acta Physiol. Scand.* **81**, 35–45, 1971.

Pelham, R. W., Vaughan, G. M., Sandock, K. L., Vaughan, M. K.: Twenty-four-hour cycle of a melatonin-like substance in the plasma of human males. *J. Clin. Endocrinol. Metab.* **37**, 341, 1973.

Perkoff, G. T., Eik-Nes, K., Nugent, C. A., et al: Studies of the diurnal variation of plasma 17-hydroxy-corticosteroids in man. *J. Clin. Endocrinol.* **19**, 432, 1959.

Peterson, J. E., Wilcox, A. A., Haley, M. I., Keith, R. A.: Hourly variation in total serum cholesterol. *Circulation* **22**, 247, 1960.

Peterson, N. T., Midgley, A. R., Jaffe, R. B.: Regulation of human gonadotropins: III. LH and FSH in sera from adult males. *J. Clin. Endocrinol.* **28**, 1473, 1968.

Pincus, G.: A diurnal rhythm in the excretion of urinary ketosteroids by young men. *J. Clin. Endocrinol.* **3**, 195, 1943.

Platen, O. V.: Über den Einfluss des Auges auf den tierischen Stoffwechsel. *Pflügers Arch.* **11**, 272, 1875.

Plotnick, L. P., Thompson, R. G., Kowarski, A., et al: Circadian variation of integrated concentration of growth hormone in children and adults. *J. Clin. Endocrinol. Metab.* **40**, 240, 1975.

Pomerat, G. R.: Cell changes in the pituitary and ovary of the white rat following exposure to constant light and darkness. *Anat. Rec.* **82**, 531, 1942.

Ponder, E., Saslow, G., Schweizer, M.: On the variations in the white-cell count of man. *Quart. J. Exp. Physiol.* **21**, 21, 1932.

Ponte, F., Ragonese, P., Albano, S. B.: Einige Aspekte der Zwischenhirn-Hypophysen-Nebennierenfunktion nach intermittierender Lichtreizung der Netzhaut. *Zbl. Ophthal.* **83**, 14, 1961.

Puntriano, G., and Meites, J.: The effects of continuous light or darkness on thyroid function in mice. *Endocrinology* **48**, 217, 1951.

Quay, W. B.: 24-hour rhythms in pineal 5-hydroxyindole-O-methyl-transferase activity in the macaque. *Proc. Soc. Exptl. Biol. Med.* **121**, 946, 1966.

Quincke, H.: Über den Einfluss des Schlafes auf die Harnabsonderung. *Arch. Exp. Path.* **7**, 115, 1877.

Quincke, H.: Über Tag- und Nachtharn. *Arch. Exp. Path.* **32**, 211, 1893.

Raab, W.: Zur Frage: Licht und Stoffwechsel des Menschen. *Z. Ges. Exp. Med.* **106**, 154, 1939.

Radnot, M.: Die Wirkung der Belichtung der Augen auf die Funktion der Gonaden. *Ophthalmologica* **127**, 422, 1954.

Radnot, M. (1961). "Neuroendokrine Beziehungen zur Ophthalmologie.'' Akadémiaí Kiadó, Budapest.

Radnot, M., and Orban, T.: Die Wirkung der Belichtung auf die sekundären sexuellen Merkmale. *Acta Med.* **3**, 1955.

Radnot, M., and Strobl, G.: Einfluss der Ausschaltung des Lichtes auf die Gonaden bei jungen Kaninchen. *Klin. Mbl. Augenheilk.* **145**, 676, 1964.

Radnot, M., and Török, E.: Die Tagesschwankungen der Eosinophilenzahl und des intraokularen Druckes. *Klin. Mbl. Augenheilk.* **130**, 763, 1957.

Radnot, M., and Wallner, E.: Periodicity in the eosinophil count in the adrenal cycle. *Ann. N.Y. Acad. Sci.* **117**, 244, 1964.

Radnot, M., and Wallner, E.: The endogenous eosinopenic reaction in different eye diseases. *Acta Ophthal.* **43**, 164, 1965.

Radnot, M., Wallner, E., Hönig, M.: Die Wirkung des Lichtes und des Hydergins auf die eosinophilen Leukozyten des Blutes. *Wiener Klin. Wschr.* **72**, 101, 1960.

Ramón y Cajal, S.: *J. Internat. Anat. et Physiol.* **8**, 337, 1891.

Ramón y Cajal, S.: Histologie du syst. nerv. de l'homme et des animaux (1911 Zit. n. R. Greving). *Dtsch. Zschr. Nervenhk.* **89**, 179, 1926.

Range, H. D.: Bevorzugte Beleuchtungsniveaus im Freien. *Lichttechnik* **23**, 356, 1971.

Rautenberg, W.: Körpergewicht und Grundumsatz beim kastrierten männlichen Vogel. *Wiss. Z. Univ. Greifswald* **2**, 229, 1952.

Reid-Hunt, B.: The influence of thyroid feeding upon poisoning by acetonitrile. *J. Biol. Chem.* **1**, 33, 1905.

Reinberg, A. (1974). Basic physiological rhythms. *In* ''Progress in Biometeorology'' (S. W. Tromp, ed.), p. 261. Swets & Zeitlinger, Amsterdam.

Reinberg, A., Apfelbaum, M., Assan, R., Lacatis, D. (1974). Persisting circadian rhythm in insulin, glucagon, cortisol etc. of healthy young women during caloric restriction (protein diet). *In* ''Chronobiology'' (L. Scheving et al, eds.), p. 88. G. Thieme, Stuttgart.

Reiter, R. J.: The effects of pineal grafts, pinealectomy and denervation of the pineal gland on the reproductive organs of male hamsters. *Neuroendocrinology* **2**, 138, 1967.

Reiter, R. J.: Pineal function in long-term blinded male and female golden hamsters. *Gen. Comp. Endocrinol.* **12**, 460, 1969.

Reiter, R. J.: Evidence for refractoriness of the pituitary-gonadal axis to the pineal gland in golden hamsters and its possible implications in annual reproductive rhythms. *Anat. Rec.* **173**, 365, 1972a.

Reiter, R. J.: Surgical procedures involving the pineal gland which prevent gonadal degeneration in adult male hamsters. *Ann. Endocrinol.* **33**, 571, 1972b.

Reiter, R. J.: Evidence for pineal-induced seasonal changes in reproductive physiology of male hamsters kept under natural environmental conditions. *Fed. Proc.* **32**, 219, 1973a.

Reiter, R. J.: Pineal control of a seasonal reproductive rhythm in male golden hamsters exposed to natural daylight and temperature. *Endocrinology* **92**, 423, 1973b.

Reiter, R. J., Blum, K., Wallace, J. E., Merritt, J. H.: Effect of the pineal gland on alcohol consumption by congenitally blind male rats. *Quart. J. Stud. Alc.* **34**, 937, 1973.

Relkin, R.: Pineal function relation to absolute darkness and sexual maturation. *Am. J. Physiol.* **213**, 999, 1967.

Relkin, R.: Combined effects of hypothalamic lesioning and light in the advancement of puberty. *Endocrinology* **82**, 865, 1968.

Remler, O.: Untersuchungen an Blinden über die 24-Stunden-Rhythmik. *Klin. Mbl. Augenheilk.* **113**, 116, 1948.

Renbourn, E. T.: Variation, diurnal and over longer periods of time, in blood haemoglobin, haematocrit, plasma protein, erythrocyte sedimentation rate, and blood chloride. *J. Hyg.* **45**, 455, 1947.

Retienne, K., Espinoza, A., Marx, K. H., Pfeiffer, E. F.: Über das Verhalten von ACTH und Cortisol im Blut von Normalen und von Kranken mit primärer und sekundärer Störung der Nebennierenrindenfunktion. *Klin. Wschr.* **43**, 205, 1965.

Ringeon, A. R.: Effects of continuous green and red light illumination on gonadal response in the English sparrow *Passer domesticus* (Linnaeus). *Am. J. Anat.* **71**, 99, 1942.

Rohles, F. H. (1969). ''Circadian Rhythms in Nonhuman Primates.'' S. Karger Verlag, Basel.

Romijn, H. J.: Structure and innervation of the pineal gland of the rabbit, *Oryctolagus cuniculus* (L.), with some functional considerations. A light and electron-microscopic investigation. *Biol. Thesis,* Free Univ. Amsterdam, Nooy, Puemerend, 1972.

Romijn, H. J.: Parasympathetic innervation of the rabbit pineal gland. *Brain Res.* **55**, 431, 1973.

Roth, W. D.: Comments on J. A. Kapper's review and observations on pineal activity. *Am. Zool.* **4**, 53, 1964.

Rowan, W.: Relation of light to bird migration and development changes. *Nature* **115**, 494, 1925.

Rowan, W.: On photoperiodism, reproductive periodicity and the annual migration of birds and certain fishes. *Proc. Boston S. Nat. Hist.* **38**, 147, 1926.

Rowan, W.: Reproductive rhythms in birds. *Nature* **122**, 11, 1928.

Rust, C. C., and Meyer, R. K.: Hair color, molt and testis size in male short-tailed weasels treated with melatonin. *Science* **165**, 921, 1969.

Sabin, F. R., Cunningham, R. S., Doan, C. A., Kindwall, J. A.: The normal rhythm of the white blood cells. *Bull. Hopkins Hosp.* **37**, 14, 1925.

Saller, K.: Probleme um die Akzeleration. *Münch. Med. Wschr.* **103**, 1263, 1961.

Saltarelli, C. G.: Light: The forgotten parameter. *Newsletter Center Light Res.* **6** (1), 1, 1977.

Santo, E.: Die histologischen Grundlagen der Reid-Hunt-Reaktion an der Schilddrüse der weissen Maus. *Z. Ges. Exp. Med.* **93**, 793, 1934.

Sayler, A., and Wolfson, A.: Role of the eyes and superior cervical ganglia on the effects of light on the pineal and gonads of the Japanese quail. *Arch. Anat.* **51**, 613, 1968a.

Sayler, A., and Wolfson, A.: Influence of the pineal gland on gonadal maturation in the Japanese quail. *Endocrinology* **83**, 1237, 1968b.

Schäfer, H. E., Schäfer, A., Kreiter, H.: Untersuchungen über die tageszeitlichen Schwankungen der Phosphor- und Kalziumausscheidung im Urin. *Z. Klin. Med.* **157**, 372, 1962.

Scharrer, E.: Über ein vegetatives optisches System. *Klin. Wochenschrift* **16**, 1521–1523, 1937.

Scharrer, E.: Photo-neuro-endocrine systems: General concepts. *Ann. N. Y. Acad. Sci.* **117**, 13, 1964.

Scharrer, E., and Scharrer, B. (1963). "Neuroendocrinology." Columbia University Press, New York.

Scheving, L. E., and Pauly, J. E.: Effect of light on corticosterone levels in plasma of rats. *Am. J. Physiol.* **210**, 1112, 1966.

Schildmacher, H.: Hoden und Schilddrüse des Gartenrotschwanzes unter dem Einfluss zusätzlicher Beleuchtung im Herbst und Winter. *Biol. Zbl.* **58**, 464, 1938.

Schildmacher, H.: Stoffwechselphysiologische Untersuchungen an männlichen Gartenrotschwänzen. *Biol. Zbl.* **71**, 238, 1952.

Schildmacher, H.: Physiologische Untersuchungen am Grünfinken im künstlichen Kurztag und nach "hormonaler Sterilisierung." *Biol. Zbl.* **75**, 327, 1956.

Schildmacher, H., and Rautenberg, W.: Über die Wirkung kleiner Mengen von Thyroxin auf das Körpergewicht bei Finkenvögeln. *Biol. Zbl.* **71**, 397, 1952.

Schildmacher, H., and Steubling, L.: Untersuchungen zur hormonalen Regulierung des Fettwerdens der Zugvögel im Frühjahr. *Biol. Zbl.* **71**, 272, 1952.

Schlegel, L., Stembera, Z. K., Pokorny, J.: Tagesrhythmus der Wehentätigkeit unter der Geburt. *Gynaecologia* **162**, 185–196, 1966.

Schoenenberger (1898). "Der Einfluss des Lichtes auf den tierischen Organismus." Berlin.

Schwarzstein, L., LaBorde, N. P., Aparicio, N. J., et al: Daily variations of FSH, LH and testosterone response to intravenous luteinizing-hormone-releasing factor (LRF) in normal men. *J. Clin. Endocrinol. Metab.* **40**, 313, 1975.

Seaman, G. V. F., Engel, R., Swank, R. L., Hissen, W.: Circadian periodicity in some physiochemical parameters of circulating blood. *Nature* **207**, 833, 1965.

Seibel, H. R., and Schweisthal, M. R.: Relationship between the pineal gland, other endocrine glands and reproductive organs of single and parabiosed golden hamsters. *Acta Endocrinol.* **74**, 434, 1973.

Selye, H. (1956). "The Stress of Life." McGraw-Hill, New York.

Selye, H. (1974). "Stress," J. P. Lippincott, Philadelphia–New York.

Serra, E. (1959). "Neurological Contribution to Action Mechanism of Intermittent Photic Stimulation. 4. International Congress of Electroencephalography and Clinical Neurophysiology," p. 427. Pergamon Press, London.

Seyderhelm, R.: Über einen durch ultraviolette Bestrahlung aktivierbaren, antianaemisch wirkenden Stoff im Blute. *Klin. Wschr.* **11**, 628, 1934.

Seyderhelm, R., and Goldberg, E.: Untersuchungen über die Wasserausscheidung bei orthostatischer Albuminurie. *Z. Klin. Med.* **105**, 539, 1927.

Sharp, G. W. G.: Reversal of diurnal rhythms of

water and electrolyte excretion in man. *J. Endocrinol.* **21**, 97, 1960a.

Sharp, G. W. G.: Reversal of leucocyte variations in man. *J. Endocrinol.* **21**, 107, 1960b.

Sharp, G. W. G.: The effect of light on diurnal leucocyte variations. *J. Endocrinol.* **21**, 213, 1960c.

Sharp, G. W. G., Slorach, S. A., Vipond, H. J.: Diurnal rhythms of keto- and ketogenic steroid excretion and the adaptation to changes of the activity-sleep routine. *J. Endocrinol.* **22**, 377, 1961.

Shaw, A. F. B.: The diurnal tides of the leucocytes in men. *J. Pathol.* **30**, 1, 1927.

Shimada, K., Yano, J., Oshima, S., Tonoue, T.: Effect of photic stimulation on hypothalamic electroencephalograph and thyroid activity in the chicken. *Neuroendocrinology* **12**, 142, 1973.

Shiotsuka, R. N., Reinberg, A., Ungar, F., et al: Circadian variation of norepinephrine ratio (NER) in health, sleep deprivation and schizophrenia. *Physiologist* **3**, 230, 1971.

Siegenthaler, W. (1970). "Klinische Pathophysiologie." Stuttgart.

Simenhoff, M. L.: Control of day-to-day salt excretion in man. Use of the blind subject as a model in its elucidation. *Clin. Res.* **16**, 396, 1968.

Simonnet, H., Thieblot, L., Melik, T.: Influence de l'épiphyse sur l'ovaire de la jeune rat. *Ann. d'Endocrinol.* **12**, 202, 1951.

Simpson, G. E.: Diurnal variations in the rate of urine excretion for two hour intervals: Some associated factors. *J. Biol. Chem.* **59**, 107, 1924.

Simpson, G. E.: The effect of sleep on urinary chlorides and pH. *J. Biol. Chem.* **67**, 505, 1926.

Simpson, H. W., and Lobban, M. C.: Effect of a 21-hour day on the human circadian excretory rhythms of 17-OHS and electrolytes. *Aerospace Med.* **38**, 1205, 1967.

Sirota, J. H., Baldwin, D. S., Villareal, H.: Diurnal variations of renal function in man. *J. Clin. Invest.* **29**, 187, 1950.

Sisson, T. R. C.: Phototherapie der Neugeborenen-Hyperbilirubinämie. *Fortschr. Med.* **91**, 563, 1973.

Smals, A. G. H., Kloppenborg, P. W. C., Benraad, T. J.: Diurnal plasma testosterone rhythm and the effect of short-term ACTH administration on plasma testosterone in man. *J. Clin. Endocrinol. Metab.* **38**, 608, 1974.

Smelser, G. K., Walton, A., Whetlam, E. O.:

The effect of light on ovarian activity in the rabbit. *J. Exptl. Biol.* **11**, 352, 1934.

Sollberger, A. (1965). "Biological Rhythm Research." Amsterdam, London, New York.

Sommer, C.: Über die Körpertemperatur des Neugeborenen. *Dtsch. Med. Wschr.* **6**, 605, 1880.

Sorour, M. F.: Versuche über den Einfluss von Nahrung, Licht und Bewegung auf Knochenentwicklung und endokrine Drüsen junger Ratten mit besonderer Berücksichtigung der Rachitis. *Beitr. Path. Anat.* **71**, 467, 1922/1923.

Speck, B.: Diurnal variation of serum iron and the latent iron-binding in normal adults. *Helv. Med. Acta* **34**, 231, 1967/1968.

Spode, E.: Die Beeinflussung der Formelemente des Blutes durch optische Strahlung. *Wiss. Z. Humboldt-Univ. Berlin II* **17**, (1952/1953).

Spode, E.: Untersuchungen über die Strahlenreaktion des Blutes. 1. Der Blutstatus beim Kaninchen als Test für UV-Einfluss. *Strahlentherapie* **93**, 15, 1954a.

Spode, E.: Untersuchungen über die Strahlenreaktion des Blutes. 3. Untersuchungen des Blutbildes nach UV-Bestrahlung. *Strahlentherapie* **93**, 588, 1954b.

Spode, E.: Untersuchungen über die Strahlenreaktion des Blutes. 4. Wirkungen des sichtbaren Lichtes auf das periphere Blutbild von Albinokaninchen. *Strahlentherapie* **96**, 111, 1955a.

Spode, E.: Untersuchungen über die Strahlenreaktion des Blutes. 5. Bestrahlungsversuche mit dem UV-Bereich. *Strahlentherapie* **96**, 595, 1955b.

Staub, H.: Untersuchungen über den Zuckerstoffwechsel des Menschen. *Z. Klin. Med.* **91**, 44, 1921.

Stephan, F. K., and Zucker, I.: Circadian rhythms in drinking behaviour and locomotor activity of rats eliminated by hypothalamic lesions. *Proc. Nat. Acad. Sci. USA* **69**, 1583, 1972.

Stöckli, Ch.: Zur Frage der Tagesschwankungen des Serumscholesterins. *Z. Klin. Chem.* **4**, 62, 1966.

Strieck, F.: Über experimentell erzeugten zentralen Diabetes. *Verh. Dtsch. Ges. Inn. Med.* **49**, 129, 1937.

Strobel, E., and Dorschner, H.: Zur Frage der Menstruationsverhältnisse bei blinden Frauen. *Geburtshilfe & Frauenheilk.* **16**, 1024, 1956.

Stutinsky, F.: Le réflexe "opto-pituitaire" chez

la grenouille. *Bull. Biol. France et Blge.* **73**, 385, 1939.

Surowiak, J., and Tilgner, S.: The influence of white light and darkness on the percentage composition of white blood corpuscles in the peripheral blood of the white mouse. *Acta Biol. Cracov.* **9**, 277, 1966.

Szafarczyk, A., Nougier-Soule, J., Assenmacher, I.: Diurnal locomotor and plasma corticosterone rhythms in rats living on photoperiodically lenghtened days. *Internat. J. Chronobiology* **2**, 373, 1974.

Tamarkin, L., and Goldman, B.: Effects of melatonin on the reproductive system in intact and pinealectomized hamsters. International Symposium: Pineal Gland. Jerusalem, Israel, November 14–17, 1977.

Tasca, C.: La pathomorphie des corrélations endocriniennes de la thyroide. *Rev. Roum. Endocrinol.* **9**, 371, 1972.

Taylor, A. N., and Wilson, R. W.: Electrophysical evidence for the action on the pineal gland in the rat. *Experientia* **26**, 267, 1970.

Thieblot, L., and Blaise, S.: Influence de la glande pinéale sur les gonades. *Ann. d'Endocrinol.* **24**, 270, 1963.

Thieblot, L., and Blaise, S.: Influence de la glande pinéale sur la spère génitale. *Progr. Brain Res.* **10**, 577, 1965.

Thieblot, L., Blaise, S., Alassimone, A.: Essai de caractérisation du principe anti-gonadotrope de la glande pinéale. *C.R. Soc. Biol.* **160**, 1574, 1967.

Thomas, J. B., and Pizzarello, D. J.: Blindness, biologic rhythms and menarche. *Obstet. Gynec. N.Y.* **30**, 507, 1967.

Thompson, A. P. D.: Relation of retinal stimulation to oestrus in the ferret. *J. Physiol.* **113**, 425, 1951.

Thorn, G. W., Forsham, P. H., Prunty, F. T. G., Hills, G. A.: *J. Am. Med. Assoc.* **137**, 1005, 1948.

Thorpe, D. H. (1967). Basic parameters in the reaction of ferrets to light (Grundbegriffe in der Reaktion von Frettchen auf Licht). *In* "The Effects of External Stimuli on Reproduction," Ciba Foundation Study Group No. 26. J. A. Churchill, London.

Thorpe, P. A., and Herbert, J.: An experimental study of the accessory optic system in the ferret. *J. Anat.* **118**, 376, 1974.

Thum, Ch., Laube, H., Schröder, K. E., Raptis, S., Pfeiffer, E. F.: Das kontinuierliche Blutzuckertagesprofil in Korrelation zum Seruminsulin bei idealgewichtigen und normalgewich-

tigen Stoffwechselgesunden. *Dtsch. Med. Wschr.* **100**, 1595, 1975.

Tilgner, S.: Zur Frage optico-vegetativer Effekte bei Fehlen retinaler visueller Lichtrezeptoren. *Naturwiss.* **53**, 13, 1966.

Tilgner, S.: Beziehungen zwischen Licht, Auge und Nebennierenaktivität. *Biol. Rundschau* **5**, 267, 1967.

Timonen, S., Franzas, B., Wichmann, K.: Photosensibility of the human pituitary. *Ann. Chir. Gynaecol. Fem.* **53**, 165–172, 1964.

Tixier-Vidal, A., and Assenmacher, I.: Etude des synthèses iodées thyroidiennes chez le canard pékin maintenu à température constante. Premiers résultats sur l'influence de la lumière et de l'obscurité permanentes. *C.R. Soc. Biol.* **153**, 721, 1959.

Traugott, K.: Über das Verhalten des Blutzuckerspiegels bei wiederholter und verschiedener Art eneteraler Zuckerzufuhr und dessen Bedeutung für die Leberfunktion. *Klin. Wschr.* **1**, 892, 1922.

Tromp, S. W.: Short and long periodical fluctuations in blood sedimentation rate, hemoglobin and diastolic blood pressure, observed in healthy male donors in 18 bloodbanks in the Northern and Southern Hemisphere. *J. Interdiscipl. Cycle Res.* **4**, 207, 1973.

Tromp, S. W. (1974). Meteorological effects on basic physiological systems. *In* "Progress in Biometeorology" (S. W. Tromp, ed.), p. 239. Swets & Zeitlinger, Amsterdam.

Tromp, S. W., and Bouma, J.: A study of the possible relationship between blindness of young male subjects and the excretion of 17-ketosteroids, hexosamines, sodium and urea in urine. *Rep. Biometeor. Res. Ctr.* **4**, 1, 1967.

Unshelm, J.: Individuelle, tages- und tageszeitabhängige Schwankungen von Blutbestandteilen beim Rind. 3. Mitteilung: Das Verhalten der Erythrozyten, des Hämoglobingehaltes und des Hämotokrits. *Zbl. Vet. Med.* **15**, 664, 1968.

Unshelm, J., and Hagemeister, H.: Individual diurnal and time-of-day variations in the blood constituents of cattle. *J. Interdiscipl. Cycle Res.* **2**, 283, 1971.

Vagnucci, A. H., McDonald, R. H., Drash, A. L., Wong, A. K. C.: Intradiem changes of plasma aldosterone, cortisol, corticosterone and growth hormone in sodium restriction. *J. Clin. Endocrinol. Metab.* **38**, 761, 1974.

Vanhelst, L., Van Cauter, E., Degaute, J. P., Golstein, J.: Circadian variations of serum thyrotropin levels in man. *J. Clin. Endocrinol. Metab.* **35**, 479, 1972.

Vannfalt, K. A.: Action de la lumière sur la composition du sang humain. *C.R. Soc. Biol.* **101**, 610, 1929.

Vaughan, G. M., Meyer, G. G., Reiter, R. J. (1978). Evidence for a pineal–gonad relationship in the human. *In* "Progress in Reproductive Biology: The Pineal and Reproduction" (R. J. Reiter, ed.), Vol. 3. S. Karger, Basel.

Vencenoscev, B. B.: Blutbefunde bei Polarforschern. Münch. med. Wschr. Beil. *Aktuelle Medizin* **114**, 4, 14, 15, 1972 (*Beilage Münch. Med. Wschr.* **114**, 1972); *Klin. Med. Moskva* **49**, 40, 1971.

Vernikos-Danellis, J., Leach, C. S., Winget, C. M., Rambaut, P. C., Mack, P. B.: Thyroid and adrenal cortical rhythmicity during bed rest. *J. Appl. Physiol.* **33**, 644, 1972.

Völker, H.: Über die tagesperiodischen Schwankungen einiger Lebensvorgänge des Menschen. *Pflügers Arch.* **215**, 43, 1927.

Vollrath, L., and Brabant, G.: Umweltbedingte Anpassung und Schädigung endokriner Organe. *Dtsch. Med. Wschr.* **99**, 1568, 1974.

V. Baerensprung, F.: Untersuchungen über die Temperaturverhältnisse des Foetus und des erwachsenen Menschen im gesunden und kranken Zustande. *Arch. Anat. u. Physiol. (Berlin)* 126, 1851.

V. Frisch, K.: Uber den Farbensinn der Fische. *Verh. Dtsch. Zool. Ges.* **20/21**, 122–133, 1911.

V. Schumacher-Marienfrid, S. (1939). "Jagd und Biologie." Springer, Berlin.

V. Schumann, H. J.: Fehlregulationen des Stoffwechsels als Folge von Erblindung. *Med. Klin.* **48**, 1772, 1953.

V. Schumann, H. J. (1973). Disturbances of sexual function in blind people. *In* "Int. Congress: The Sun in the Service of Mankind," B 19. Unesco-House, Paris.

V. Törne, H.: Der einfluss farbigen Lichtes auf Entwicklung und Aktivität des Kornkäfers Calandra granaria. *L.Z. Hyg. Zool.* **33**, 53–64, 1941.

Walfish, P. G., Britton, A., Melville, P. H., Ezrin, C.: A diurnal pattern in the rate of disappearance of I^{131}-labeled-1-thyroxine from the serum. *J. Clin. Endocrinol.* **21**, 582, 1961.

Walter, M. R., Martinet, L., Moret, B., Thibault, C.: Régulation photopériodique de l'activité sexuelle chez le lapin mâle et femelle. (Photopériodische Regulierung der sexuellen Aktivität beim männlichen und weiblichen Kaninchen.) *Arch. Anat.* **51**, 773–780, 1968.

Warren, D. C., and Scott, H.: Influence of light on ovulation in the fowl. *J. Exptl. Zool.* **74**, 137, 1936.

Wassner, L.: Untersuchungen bei jugendlichen Blinden als Beitrag zur vegetativen Steuerung des Stoffwechsels über die Sehbahn. *Med. Mschr.* **8**, 530, 1954.

Webster, B. R., Guansing, A. R., Paice, J. C.: Absence of diurnal variation of serum TSH. *J. Clin. Endocrinol.* **34**, 899, 1972.

Weeke, J.: Circadian variations of the serum thyrotropin level in normal subjects. *Scand. J. Clin. Lab. Invest.* **31**, 337, 1973.

Weitzman, E. D., Nogeire, C., Perlow, M., et al: Effects of a prolonged 3-hour sleep-wake cycle on sleep stages, plasma cortisol, growth hormone and body temperature in man. *J. Clin. Endocrinol. Metab.* **38**, 1018, 1974.

Westergren, A.: Die Senkungsreaktion. *Erg. Inn. Med.* **26**, 577, 1924.

Wever, R.: Autonome circadiane Periodik des Menschen unter dem Einfluss verschiedener Beleuchtungsbedingungen. *Pflügers Arch.* **306**, 71, 1969.

Wever, R.: Zur Zeitgeber-Stärke eines Licht-Dunkel-Wechsels für die circadiane Periodik des Menschen. *Pflügers Arch.* **321**, 133, 1970.

Wever, R.: Der Einfluss des Lichtes auf die circadiane Periodik des Menschen. I. Teil: Einfluss auf die autonome Periodik. *Z. Physik. Med.* **3**, 121, 1973.

Wever, R.: Der Einfluss des Lichtes auf die circadiane Periodik des Menschen. II. Teil: Zeitgeber-Einfluss. *Z. Physik. Med.* **3**, 137, 1974.

Whitaker, W. L.: Effect of light on reproductive cycle of peromysus leucopus noveboracensis. *Proc. Soc. Biol. Med.* **34**, 329, 1936.

Wilhelm, R.: Vergleichende Untersuchungen über den nervös gesteuerten Farbwechsel der Fische. *Z. Vergl. Physiol.* **65**, 153–190, 1969.

Williams, C. M.: Control of pupal diapause by the direct action of light on the insect brain. *Sciena* **140**, 386, 1963.

Williams, G. H., Cain, J. P., Dluhy, R. G., Underwood, R. H.: Study of the control of plasma aldosterone concentration in normal man. I. Response to posture, acute and chronic volume depletion and sodium loading. *J. Clin. Invest.* **51**, 1731, 1972.

Wilson, W. O.: Photocontrol of oviposition in gallinaceus birds. *Ann. N.Y. Acad. Sci.* **117**, 94–203, 1964.

Wimmer, A. (1856). "Der Einfluss der Erblindung in der Kindheit auf die Entwicklung des

Körpers, auf das Gemüt und den Geist.'' *Jahresber. Königl. Blindenanstalt,* München, 1856.

Wisser, H., Doerr, P., Stamm, D., et al: Tagesperiodik der Ausscheidung von Elektrolyten, Katecholamin-Metaboliten und 17-Hydroxycorticosteroiden im Harn. *Klin. Wschr.* **51**, 242, 1973.

Wolfson, A., and Turek, F. W.: Melatonin and the photoperiodic gonadal cycle in birds. International Symposium: Pineal Gland. Jerusalem, Israel, November 14–17, 1977.

Wolstenholme, G. E. W., and Knight, J. (1971). "The Pineal Gland." Ciba Foundation Symposium. Edinburgh, London.

Wolstenholme, G. E. W., and Maeve O'Connor, B. A. (1967). "The Effects of External Stimuli on Reproduction." J. A. Churchill, London.

Wurtman, R. J. (1966). "Catecholamines." Little, Brown, Boston, Massachusetts.

Wurtman, R. J.: Effects of light and visual stimuli on endocrine function. *Neuroendocrinology* **2**, 20, 1967.

Wurtman, R. J.: The pineal and endocrine function. *Hosp. Prac.* **4**, 32–37, 1969.

Wurtman, R. J. (1971). Summary of symposium. *In* "The Pineal Gland". (G. E. W. Wolstenholme and J. Knight, eds.), p. 379. Ciba Foundation Symposium, Edinburgh, London.

Wurtman, R. J., Altschulte, M. D., Holmgren, U.: Effects of pinealectomy and of bovine pineal extracts in rats. *Am. J. Physiol.* **197**, 108, 1959.

Wurtman, R. J., Axelrod, J., Chu, E. W., Fisher, E. J.: Mediation of some effects of illumination on the rat estrous cycle by the sympathetic nervous system. *Endocrinology* **75**, 266, 1964a.

Wurtman, R. J., Axelrod, J., Fisher, J. E.: Melatonin synthesis in the pineal gland: Effects of light mediated by the sympathetic nervous system. *Science* **143**, 1328, 1964b.

Wurtman, R. J., Axelrod, J., Kelly, D. E. (1968). "The Pineal." Academic Press, New York.

Wurtman, R. J., Axelrod, J., Phillips, L. S.: Melatonin synthesis in the pineal gland, control by light. *Science* **142**, 1071–1073, 1963.

Wurtman, R. J., Roth, W., Altschulte, M. D., Wurtman, J. J.: Interactions of the pineal and exposure to continuous light on organ weight of female rats. *Acta Endocrinol.* **36**, 617, 1961.

Wurtman, R. J., and Weisel, J.: Environmental lighting and neuroendocrine function: Relationship between spectrum of light source and gonadal growth. *Endocrinology* **85**, 1218, 1969.

Yalow, R. S., Varsano-Aharon, N., Echemendia, E., Berson, S. A.: HGH and ACTH secretory responses to stress. *Hor. Metab. Res.* **1** (1), 1969.

Yano, K.: A comparative study on the growth in height and weight of normal, blind and deaf school-children. *Kurume Med. J.* **1**, 71, 1954.

Young, J. Z.: *J. Exp. Biol.* **12**, 254, 1935.

Zacharias, L., and Wurtman, R. J.: Blindness: Its relation to age of menarche. *Science* **144**, 1154–1155, 1964.

Zacharias, L., and Wurtmann, R. J.: Age at menarche. *New Engl. J. Med.* **280**, 668, 1969a.

Zacharias, L., and Wurtmann, R. J.: Blindness and menarche. *Obstet. Gynecol.* **33**, 603, 1969b.

Zicha, L., and Ali, B. S.: Über den Einfluss von Koffein auf den Tagesrhythmus der Vanillinmandelsäure, Vanillinsäure und Homovanillinsäure. *Med. Welt.* **30**, 1674, 1969.

Author Index*

*Numbers in italics refer to pages on which complete references are listed.

Subject Index